The Truth
about
Breast Implants

The Truth about Breast Implants

Randolph H. Guthrie, M.D.
with Doug Podolsky

Foreword by Betty Rollin,
author of *First You Cry*

A ROBERT L. BERNSTEIN BOOK

JOHN WILEY & SONS, INC.
New York • Chichester • Brisbane • Toronto • Singapore

Library of Congress Cataloging-in-Publication Data:

Guthrie, Randolph H.
    The truth about breast implants / Randolph H. Guthrie
with Doug Podolsky.
      p.   cm.
    Includes index.
    ISBN 0-471-59418-0 (acid-free paper)
    1. Breast implants. I. Podolsky, Doug M., 1957–   . II. Title.
RD539.8.G883 1993
618.1'9059—dc20   93-13677

Printed in the United States of America

10 9 8 7 6 5 4 3 2 1

This book is for my wife, Beatrice.

List of Trade Names

Ivalon is a trademark of Elizabeth J. Melaragno

Teflon is a registered trademark of E.I. DuPont de Nemours and Company

Dacron is a registered trademark of E.I. DuPont de Nemours and Company

Même is a registered trademark of Medical Engineering Corporation

Jell-O is a registered trademark of General Foods Corporation

Silastic is a registered trademark of Dow Corning Corporation

Replicon is a registered trademark of Medical Engineering Corporation

MISTI GOLD is a trademark of Bioplasty, Inc.

Bio-Oncotic is a trademark of Bioplasty, Inc.

Important Notice

This book has been written as a general reference guide for women who have had or are considering having breast implants, but by no means should this book be considered as a substitute for professional medical advice. The reader is urged to consult with her own physician, as no one course of treatment is right for everyone.

While every effort has been made to provide accurate and authoritative information, the authors and publisher assume no responsibility or liability for any error or omission, or any outcome from using the materials contained in this book.

PREFACE

There is no need to fear breast enlargement or reconstruction. These are very safe, relatively painless, uncomplicated, and very satisfying procedures when a saline-filled implant is used. Some of my colleagues have undermined women's confidence in these procedures by using silicone gel–filled implants, which are dangerous, and by performing operations that are too complicated and too risky. For years, I have written professional articles and lectured about the dangers of these practices to no avail. Finally, I became so angry at the way the truth was being withheld from women that I decided to write this book. I find these activities medically and ethically indefensible and feel that it's time someone gave women the true story—so that each woman can make the best informed decision for herself.

The doctors who refused to listen to the warnings are presently being severely criticized for their misdeeds and will soon be called before the bar of justice to explain them. It is difficult to feel any sympathy for them because they have known well for some time that what they have been doing has hurt many women. They have arrogantly ignored all warnings, and are still unrepentant.

As a result, many women have been directly injured and countless others discouraged from achieving the self-improvement that might have greatly bettered their self-esteem and their lives. It is to those women who think they have no viable alternatives that I address my message. You can have restored or larger breasts without fear. I hope that when you are finished reading this book, you will understand the options and agree with me.

I have tried for some 15 years now to convince plastic surgeons that silicone gel–filled breast implants are too risky and that they should switch to implants filled with harmless saline—sterile saltwater. Just why so many doctors would not listen has always been a mystery to me. At times, I feared that I must be crazy. How could I be right and so many others be wrong? They seemed to be in mass denial. Even when the FDA raised serious questions about health risks from silicone gel–filled implants, the American Society of Plastic and Reconstructive Surgeons, the professional umbrella organization, spent more time covering up and safeguarding the profession against lawsuits than it did trying to arrive at the truth about silicone gel–filled implants. For its part, the society says that with new leadership the society has changed its ways. Only time will tell. What's clear is that at the first inkling that federal authorities were going to scrutinize gel-filled implants, the society began amassing a war chest and initiated a huge lobbying effort to fight any regulatory oversight (see Chapter 4). Concomitantly, the society certainly has done nothing to promote the use of the safe saline-filled implants.

The society isn't finished lobbying. Through its misguided efforts it has even managed to get the FDA to knuckle under and rewrite the "informed consent" documents given to patients who choose to take part in studies of silicone gel–filled implants. Incredible as it may sound, the society has convinced the FDA itself to downplay the full extent of what is known about the risks of silicone gel–filled implants, including, for instance, the possibility of birth defects in offspring of women with silicone gel–filled implants.

No one enjoys incurring the wrath of fellow members of a club. No one, including me, likes to be the one pointing the finger at colleagues. However, I finally became convinced that I had to write this book and clear my own conscience by making a maximum effort to arm women with the facts so they can make the safest choices.

It seems that everyone—implant makers to plastic surgeons, and even the FDA—has had something vital to hide from the American public. As a result most Americans still don't know the full extent of the possible risks of silicone gel–filled implants. This book tries to bridge the information gap by explaining in plain language things about implants most plastic surgeons don't tell their patients. It reveals outrageous details that manufacturers of silicone gel–filled breast implants would rather have kept secret. These are details that even the FDA doesn't want Americans to know: the truth, for instance, about the FDA's complicity in allowing manufacturers to market silicone gel–filled implants year after year even though it suspected that there were serious risks and that adequate safety studies had never been done.

What concerns and outrages me most about this information gap is that many women have been left with the notion that there are no safe ways to enlarge small breasts or replace breasts lost to cancer surgery. The coverage by major newspapers of restrictions placed on silicone gel–filled implants by the FDA typically makes no mention of the option of saline-filled implants or else glosses over their availability. There was practically no information aired about saline-filled implants even during the days and weeks after the FDA's decision, when you would expect some in-depth pieces about women's options to appear in the media. Typical was one article in *USA TODAY* that offered over 1,000 words about women's anxieties over silicone gel–filled implants and only 100 words about alternatives such as saline-filled implants and tissue transplant surgery.

More recently, in writing about the dangers of silicone gel–filled breast implants, the press erroneously tarred saline-filled implants with the same brush. For example, an article in the February 4, 1993, issue of *The Wall Street Journal*, titled "Saline Implants Appear to Carry Hazards as Well," reported that California investigators had found that the "presence of any implant, silicone or saline, impedes mammography . . . by 30 percent to 50 percent." This is simply not true. The investigators from the Breast Center in Van Nuys, California, never even looked at simple saline-filled implants; they looked at double-lumen implants, which have an inner envelope of silicone gel, and polyurethane foam–covered implants, which are gel-filled. The truth, in my opinion, is that saline-filled implants, though unfairly scathed by association in recent events, are safe and are the best option for women who want implants. I will explain my position in this book so that you can make the best choice for yourself.

In the following pages I will try to suggest ways to find a surgeon who is truly knowledgeable about breast augmentation and reconstruction. I also explain in understandable language just what you can expect, step by step, during breast enlargement and reconstruction surgery as well as what you need to know about mammography afterward.

Implants are not the only options that doctors may offer you, so I've included a chapter on the fascinating—and sometimes downright dangerous—surgeries in which breasts are fashioned out of a patient's own body tissues. I don't recommend these, as I'll explain in detail in Chapter 3. After 20 years of performing breast surgery exclusively, I have come to the conclusion that the simplest operations not only are the quickest and safest but also give the best results. It is my hope that this book will help you find the simplest solutions for your needs and give you the information you need to have confidence that you are making the best possible choice.

ACKNOWLEDGMENTS

I am indebted to Dolly Broad for relating her story in this book; to Irene Ladden, R.N., my long-time nurse; to Susan Simmons, my assistant for 23 years; to Betty Rollin for her friendship and the Foreword to this book; to Reuven Snyderman, M.D., my mentor and predecessor as chief of plastic surgery at Memorial Sloan-Kettering Cancer Center; to Bob Bernstein who enticed me into writing this book; and to those few, stubborn colleagues who have, through the years, steadfastly refused to use silicone gel even when patients ended up going elsewhere for their surgery.

CONTENTS

Epilogue: Putting It All in Perspective: The Decline of Ethics and the Need for Responsibility 119

The Attitude Problem / Falling Standards / Take Charge

Appendix: Contacts for Additional Information 127

Index 139

FOREWORD

My first prosthesis was a sock. It belonged to my (then) husband. It was too big, and I soon moved on to pantyhose. Next I tried a hospital handout: a nylon-covered wad of Dacron that I safety-pinned to the inside of my bra. There were two problems. First, even if I didn't move my left arm, which I tried not to, the thing was weightless and rode up. Second, it didn't have a nipple. The first problem was the real one, but I became obsessed with the second. I began a serious hunt for a nipple. My search led me to a notions store, where I perused the buttons. Many were nipple-sized, but they were too hard. Undefeated, I moved on to the fringe counter. (You know, fringes, ball fringes, that which hangs from cheap bedspreads in motels.) As an elderly saleswoman with a permanent wave watched, I gave one of the balls a little feel. Perfect. I'm a tightwad now and was a tightwad then and would have liked to buy one ball. But the minimum purchase was a quarter of a yard. Still, it was a good deal: eight nipples for twenty-five cents. (This was 1975. Today, they'd probably be a dollar twenty-five or something outrageous like that.)

So now I had two little nipples sticking out, the real one and the ball of the ball fringe, which I had sewn on the nylon pad. But I had not solved the ride-up problem; ten minutes after insertion, the newly nippled pad would wind up in the neighborhood of my neck.

The Truth about Breast Implants

Get serious, I told myself, and I did. I found out about a made-to-order prostheses maker who worked out of a basement of the Medical Center of the University of Michigan. Mr. Lee was his name, an engaging young man whose prosthesis making involved taking the same kind of impression dentists take—only you are the tooth. I sat in a chair (which resembled a dentist's chair) stripped to the waist, and Mr. Lee dipped into a large bowl filled with a substance that looked like overcooked oatmeal and, with a plastic spatula, smeared it over the flat part of my chest. I remember it was cold. He poured some other stuff over me, then wrapped me in gauze. When the entire mess had hardened and I was beginning to have second thoughts about Mr. Lee and wonder if anyone would hear me scream, he ripped the thing off my body, explaining that this was a "negative" from which a prosthesis would come. Indeed it did. Two weeks later a box arrived, and in it was what I less-than-affectionately came to call The Blob.

I'll say this for The Blob: it didn't ride up. But that's all I'll say for it. It was heavy. It was hot. In the summer it stuck to me like algae. I moved on. By now—1977 or so—there were nicer blobs on the market. I tried this one, I tried that one. They were all hot and heavy. I thought about reconstruction, but I didn't want more surgery, and I didn't get a sense that the result would be good. So I endured the blobs and in the summer occasionally went braless and taped the nylon pad directly onto my skin, which sort of worked, except that I'd occasionally stand up and find it on the floor.

In 1983 I had a second mastectomy. Now I needed two blobs. Misery. I tried a padded bra and sewed in weights. Better than two blobs; still, it felt like a harness. Sometimes

Foreword

I said the hell with it and didn't wear anything, but even in loose clothing, from a side view, I sort of disappeared.

The time had come for implants.

I'd like to say I did some intelligent research, found out that saline was the way to go, and chose Dr. Guthrie because he used saline. The truth is I wasn't smart. I was lucky. I had a smart friend, Marilyn Snyder, who was my classmate at Sarah Lawrence. She had also had two mastectomies and had written a book about implants (An Informed Decision). In her book she did not say who her own surgeon was, but I wheedled it out of her. I figured she'd done the research; she'd know who'd be good. And she did.

In 1985 I became the new owner of two lovely, soft, untroublesome saline-filled breast implants. No more weights, no more hot plastic sticking to the skin, no more, "Oh dear, it was here a minute ago." And hear this: they stay up by themselves! No more harness, no more bra! And far more important than any of that: no worry. I now know that even if they leak, it's only water. (I did have a capsular contracture—a slight hardening—with one of the implants, but this was surgically corrected in a brief procedure with local anesthesia, and the problem never returned.)

I'm happy with my good fortune, but I'm angry that more women haven't had the same good fortune. The Truth about Breast Implants should change that. I fervently hope it does. Happiness loves company, too.

Betty Rollin
Author of First, You Cry

1

∾

The Quest for Perfect Breasts

The Grand Illusion

Like you, I have read dozens of news stories about the Food and Drug Administration's (FDA's) clampdown on silicone gel–filled breast implants. Most convey the impression that women now must enroll in strictly enforced, government-sanctioned clinical studies if they wish to have their breasts rebuilt after cancer surgery or enlarged.

Nothing could be further from the truth.

Both procedures are still available in the United States to any woman who needs them. But instead of becoming a human guinea pig in silicone gel studies, a woman can choose to have breast implants filled with harmless saline— sterile saltwater. The fact that so many credible news organizations have missed or downplayed such a big part of the story makes me wonder whether my colleagues in the plastic surgery community have been truly forthcoming with information about alternatives. As a result, the public is now under the mistaken impression that all breast implants are risky.

They're not. Only silicone gel–filled implants have been linked with an ever-growing list of debilitating disorders, corporate shenanigans, and medical high jinks. In the wake of the FDA's hearings, saline-filled implants have been left unscathed. That's comforting news for millions of women with very small or mismatched breasts as well as for those with breast cancer, for whom the loss of a breast can be emotionally devastating.

For better or worse, we still live in a society where breasts are perceived as a woman's sign of sexuality, of motherhood, of nurturing. Doctors have long been willing to help women have larger breasts. Since early in this century, doctors have been reaching into their black bags and pulling out an astonishing array of substances to inject and implant behind the breast to create a larger, rounder bosom. Through surgical hocus-pocus, doctors are even taking tissue from the abdomen and buttock and reshaping it as breasts to replace those lost to cancer. Everything from paraffin wax, body fat, and straight silicone injections to ocean sponge implants have been touted. In the past, as today, the assurances patients received about the safety of the procedures sometimes turned out to be the grandest illusion of all.

Shots in the Dark

For more than a century, breast enlargement and restoration methods have been devised not through standardized scientific methods but on an apparently whimsical trial-and-error basis. Recalling the often bizarre history of breast augmentation and restoration helps put today's headlines in perspective. It will not always be possible to stick to strict chronological order, however, because of overlapping events. The story begins in 1912, when, only ten years after doctors first proposed using paraffin wax injections to enlarge women's breasts, reports of hard lumps, inflammation, and even cancer began to appear. But doctors, and even entrepreneurial laypeople, continued doing wax injections. Reports of hard masses and late complications, some requiring mastectomy or breast removal to correct, were still cropping up in the medical journals even into the 1950s and 1960s.

That's when doctors turned to injections of liquid silicone, a compound that was believed to be 100 percent inert, meaning that it would not cause reactions in the body. Today, it is clear that nothing is completely inert and that, at the very least, fibrous capsules of scar tissue will grow around any implant made of foreign material. Silicone shots were a disaster, and the procedure itself involved much more than the term "shots" suggests. Surgeons first had to make an incision below the breast and open up enough underlying tissue to make a pocket behind the breast. Surgeons would then insert a long, narrow tube into the pocket and close the incision. Only then could they shoot liquid silicone through the tube to fill the pocket and make the breast look larger. Problems often cropped up during the procedure. The silicone was so viscous that very often it would not go through the tube easily. So the doctor would have to use a hand piston with a heavy spring much like a caulking gun. Or the surgical team would have to resort to a device with a foot pedal, which sometimes required the weight of two people to force silicone behind the breast.

Ironically, silicone "shots" led to the same complications as did paraffin injections. Inevitably, scar tissue would form, and frequently some of the liquid silicone would escape, and migrate throughout the body, and form little lumps. Not only did the lumps look and feel bad, they were indistinguishable from tumors. In an effort to prevent the liquid silicone from migrating, Japanese practitioners came up with a clever idea, which proved to be too clever. They mixed olive oil (a known irritant) with the liquid silicone. In reaction the body very quickly produced heavy scar tissue around the liquid silicone—olive oil mixture which kept it in place. The problem, of course, was that the results produced breasts as hard as rock. Horrified patients would have to undergo mastectomies in order to remove the mess. In the mid-1970s, Dow Corning stopped deliveries of liquid silicone in the United States. Yet even after that, some plastic surgeons stripped the covers off the first silicone gel—filled implants and pumped the gel directly into the breast. But more about implants later.

Fat and Flap Transplants

As soon as problems with liquid silicone arose, doctors began experimenting with what seemed to be almost certainly safe: injections and transplants of a patient's own fat from the abdomen or buttock. Unfortunately, it didn't work. As doctors were surprised to discover, in many cases the body simply reabsorbed the fat or the fat liquefied and scarred, leading to misshapen breasts. Plastic surgeons also tried shaping existing breast tissues into cone shapes, but the results were often disappointing because of the seemingly obvious limitations in the amount of buildup possible, especially in women who were small breasted to begin with.

Teams of doctors who specialized in reconstructing breasts lost to cancer began experimenting with the notion of fashioning a new breast out of transplanted flaps of muscle and fat from the abdomen and buttock. This method, which was first tried in 1982, has been dubbed the "Rolls Royce method" because it is elegant but unnecessarily complex. It would be more aptly named the "Corvair method" because the complication rate, including death, is so high that it's impossible to believe that it is worth the risk. Such tissue transplants have not been adopted for breast enlargement. Still, efforts aimed at transferring tissue from one part of the body to the breast continue, as you'll learn in Chapter 3.

From Sponge Implants to Bubble-Wrap

In the mid-1950s, surgeons began experimenting with implants made of natural sponges from the ocean. Not surprisingly, patients' immune systems rejected them. So doctors then tried synthetic sponges, made of polyvinyl alcohol, which were called "Ivalon™" sponges. In 1958, buoyed by studies with mice as well as patients who had Ivalon implants in their skulls following head-cancer surgery, two doctors from Johns Hopkins University in Baltimore published a paper describing the implantation of the sponges into 32 women for breast enlargement. After several years of follow-up, the doctors announced that there were very few complications and no evidence of tumor formation. However, they concluded that "the final chapter in the use of this material cannot be told for a number of years." And they warned that every patient must be clearly appraised of the newness of the method and the possibility of being recalled to the hospital at some future time for removal of the implants if any tissue reactions developed. "Any surgeon not willing to shoulder this responsibility," they wrote, "should probably not use the material on patients with a long life-expectancy."

Many plastic surgeons jumped on the procedure. But, although Ivalon sponges did not cause dramatic reactions in the body, they did eventually cause the body to grow fibrous scar tissue, which entered into all the holes of the sponge. When the scar tissue eventually contracted, the baseball-sized sponges eventually transformed into the size of large marbles and became just as hard. In 1955, doctors thought of surrounding the sponge with a polyethylene sac to keep out scar tissue. But the infection rate was too high, and the final chapter of the Ivalon implant was soon written—and discarded.

Among the other types of short-lived synthetic sponges developed and implanted into women was one that looked like a ball of bubble wrap. In theory, it probably would have worked. The implants were full of air and compressible, and women said they were quite pleased. The problem was that reports started to come in that when the breasts were squeezed, a few of the cells would break with a loud pop! The same thing would sometimes happen during plane travel when ascending. There was also a high rate of infection and extrusion, meaning that the implants would wear against the breast and finally break through the skin. Because of those problems, doctors finally threw up their hands and threw out

The Quest for Perfect Breasts

sponges of all types, which, by the end, included one that was coated with nonstick Teflon®.

Silicone Gel–Filled Implants

Then, in 1965, Dow Corning made available the "Silastic®" silicone gel–filled implant, invented in 1962 by Dr. Thomas Cronin in Houston. The story goes that, one evening, one of Dr. Cronin's residents, Dr. Frank Gerow, was carrying a plastic bag filled with blood to a patient and remarked to Dr. Cronin that the bag felt remarkably like a breast. Dr. Cronin gave the transfusion bag a squeeze and had to agree. Cronin sent Gerow to talk to executives at Dow Corning in Midland, Michigan, which at the time was just entering the medical field. Among those who helped fashion the first implant was Dr. Silas Braley, a doctor knowledgeable about silicone-rubber chemistry. The first silicone sacs were filled with saline—sterile saltwater—but they broke in a clinical trial. Later studies with sacs filled with silicone gel were deemed successful. That unfortunate experience with the very first saline-filled breast implant set the stage for the medical mindset for decades to come. It would not be until the early 1970s that saline-filled, or inflatable, implants were made commercially available.

Problems Emerge

Fortunately, paraffin and silicone injections and the various sponges were common before my time, so I was able to avoid temptation. My main experience began after I became chief of plastic surgery at Memorial Sloan-Kettering Cancer Center in 1971, when I began to use Dow Corning's Cronin implant. At the time it seemed to be a marvel. It was a silicone rubber envelope filled with soft, silicone gel that felt like very thick jelly. For the first time, breasts of cancer patients could be reconstructed successfully. Patients who wanted larger breasts flocked to the offices of plastic surgeons. And, although a significant percentage of implants became hard, patients were mostly ecstatic, particularly considering the methods that had been available previously. And when patients were happy, most doctors felt little need to follow them closely.

Soon silicone gel–filled implants were being manufactured in all types of designs and implanted using all sorts of techniques. Implants were available in high- or low-profile styles and in round, oval, or teardrop shapes; and some, including a variety that I was among the first to use and eventually reject, had polyurethane coverings. There were even some implants designed with Dacron® patches on their backs to help anchor them in the body. Most turned out to be bad ideas, as I'll show in more detail in Chapter 4. Surgeons would slip the implants into surgically crafted pockets behind the breast through incisions made either across the nipple, around the nipple, under the fold of the breast, under the armpit or, if a tummy lift was being done at the same time, through a surgically created tunnel starting from a bikini-line incision at the stomach.

Eventually, a majority of the implanted breasts became hard. Doctors discovered that it was not the implant that had hardened but, in virtually all women, a capsule of thick scar tissue that had formed around the implant and had tightened

The Quest for Perfect Breasts

up. The "capsule," as it's called, can be likened to a golf ball: the center is rubber, but when it has a tight cover surrounding it, it feels rock-hard. When the capsules in women became mildly tight, the breasts became very firm; when the capsules became severely tight, women looked disfigured. As their scar tissue contracted, it tended to take the shape of a sphere, the upper curve of which became visible in the upper part of the breast. Instead of having a teardrop shape, the breasts would bulge out on top, giving a very unnatural "Barbie doll" appearance. The result could also be very painful if the surrounding tissue were drawn in to the center of the twisting mass of capsular scar tissue. This is particularly true with women who undergo mastectomy, or breast removal surgery, after which there is a good deal of scar tissue on the chest and up under the arm.

In large studies with silicone gel–filled breast implants, between 60 and 90 percent of women experienced some degree of "capsular contracture," as the condition is called. At first, doctors were baffled. Women went back into surgery, and the scar tissue capsules were either cracked open or removed or softened with injections of steroid. Doctors would often find the implants ruptured and discover evidence of calcification, especially if the implants had been in place for a long time.

Frustrated doctors pounced on the dubious concept of bursting the capsules without surgery by squeezing the breasts with sheer manual pressure. Believe it or not, doctors dreamed up the technique after caring for a woman who discovered that one of her firm breast implants softened after she was hugged and squeezed very tightly by a professional football player at a party and heard a loud pop. When she ran to the bathroom and examined herself, she said, she found that the breast that had been squeezed was soft. Her doctors published the story in the journal *Plastic and Reconstructive Surgery*.

Soon, in doctors' offices everywhere, physicians were squeezing patients' hardened breasts with all their might to break up their capsules. The technique, however, did not solve the hardness problem. Often, the procedure did not break the capsule and therefore was useless. And it was usually exceedingly painful. When it did work, not only did implants almost always get hard again in a few days or weeks, but if the capsule was not completely broken up, the breast would look misshapen. Internal bleeding and bruises frequently resulted, sometimes extending all the way down the side of the body. At worst, the pressure would rupture the implant, bursting silicone gel into surrounding muscle and fat. Reports began to appear of silicone gel oozing out of the nipple following the procedure and of hard nodules of silicone, called granulomas, appearing on women's chests. Still, the importance of that was largely lost on doctors in the early days. Unbelievably, some papers focused not on the risk to women but on the possibility that surgeons' thumb joints could be dislocated as a result of pushing too hard to break the capsule.

Staying Soft

Doctors are still trying to figure out how to prevent implants from becoming hard. Some have tried using steroids or antibiotics around the implants or in them. Steroids inside the implant seem to help. Care is required because using it outside the implant or adding too much inside tends to thin the skin of the breast, leading to stretch marks and even making it easier for implants to break through. Antibiotics don't seem to do anything. The most ludicrous "solution" to the hardness problem came in the late 1970s, when doctors doing breast enlargements began placing implants behind the pectoral, or chest, muscle. The original proponents of this idea claimed that capsules could not tighten up because they would bond to and be held open by the ribs. Even if they did get tight, they said, the thickness and softness of the overlying muscles would disguise their hardness and spherical shape.

Unfortunately, it has since become clear that implants placed against the lining of the ribs form scar tissue that can bind chest muscle to the bones, leading to a loss of arm motion and severe "pulling" pains. What's more, the capsular scar tissue that forms is so strong that it can rip away from the rib lining anyway, leading to painful tightening. The muscle, being less than one-quarter of an inch thick, is totally unable to disguise these deficiencies. It even ruins good results because overlying muscle tends to flatten implants. In fact, one of the major proponents of the under-the-muscle procedure later claimed that the best results were possible only when a heavy capsule formed, because only then did the implant push forward enough to make the breast look natural.

When I first heard all this at a medical conference, I stood up and said, "Now, we've come full circle in the whole process of controlled, programmed lunacy." In my opinion, implants are justifiably placed against the lining of the ribs only after a mastectomy because the breast is missing, and the remaining skin is too thin to hold the implant. It is something to be avoided in purely cosmetic breast enlargements. But these colleagues have been so intent on using silicone gel–filled implants that they are prepared to seize any idea that will justify their continued use. They need to believe that putting the implant under the muscle will solve all their problems. They refuse to turn to the saline-filled implant, which has always been the real solution.

The Return of Saline-Filled Implants

It wasn't until the mid-1970s that surgeons, discouraged by their inability to prevent implants from hardening, began to take another look at saline-filled implants, which by that time had become commercially available. Clinical studies were beginning to show that there was a lower incidence of capsular contracture using saline implants compared to gel-filled implants, though it was unclear why. The problem remained, however, that the saline-filled implants leaked in unacceptable numbers, causing breasts to deflate. Fortunately, saline is only sterile saltwater, which is harmlessly absorbed by the body.

The cause of the leakage problem in early implants, it turns out, was often the design of the valve, the technique of underfilling the implants, and the body's amazing ability to siphon saltwater out of the implants, as you'll learn in Chapter 5. These problems were ultimately solved, bringing the rate of leaking implants in my experience down to an acceptable less than one percent. In retrospect, it seems that only those of us who specialized almost exclusively in breast plastic surgery recognized the potential of saline implants. We developed techniques that, along with improved designs, minimized the leakage problem. Doctors who did only a small percentage of breast surgery had their minds set against saline-filled implants because of the early failure rate and stuck with silicone gel–filled implants, which did not visibly deflate even if millions of silicone molecules were being spewed undetectably into the body.

Silicone Spinoffs

In January 1978, the journal *Science* reported electron microscopy studies that proved what any alert plastic surgeon had known all along: that silicone did indeed sweat, or "bleed," through the silicone envelope. Surgeons operating on patients with hardened silicone implants had become accustomed to finding the sticky silicone stuck on the outside of intact, unbroken gel-filled implants. Manufacturers tried several redesigns in attempts to overcome the problem. In the mid-1980s they developed twin-compartment, or "double-lumen," implants, a hybrid consisting of an inner sac of silicone gel surrounded by an outer sac that could be filled with saline. The concept is interesting only because it was a backhanded admission on the part of the surgeons who used them that there was a serious problem with gel-filled implants, but it allowed them to continue to use the gel while mentally climbing on the saline bandwagon.

Proponents of the double-lumen implant believed that if you had two shells, you could prevent silicone gel from getting out of the implant. According to the theory, if only 1 particle of silicone gel per 100,000 gets out through the first wall and only 1 per 100,000 gets out of the second wall, only 1 particle per 10 billion would get out through both shells. The fact is that the molecules that pass the membrane are the small ones. Any molecule that crosses the first wall will then go through the second wall.

Foam-Covered Implants—The Worst

Another type of implant—one that had a fuzzy polyure-thane foam covering—was similarly based on an interesting but false theory. The idea for the new implant was based on the observation that scar tissue fibers in contracted capsules line up in parallel instead of at random, as scar tissue normally does. The inventor thought that the rough polyurethane on the implant might trap the scar tissue fibers as they were laid down at random, preventing them from lining up so they could not become as tight.

This implant was not the result of years of testing by a major laboratory. It was the brainchild of a man whom we will call the "inventor-peddler" who bought silicone gel–filled implants and affixed to their surface a layer of polyurethane.

In the mid-1970s, he hooked up with a prominent plastic surgeon whom we will call the "doctor-promoter." He lent his name to the product and put it in his patients. He gave talks at medical meetings about how great the implant was and wrote an article in a major journal suggesting that it solved the problem of capsular contracture.

At that time, a few of us at Memorial Sloan-Kettering Cancer Center were trying to perfect a way to reconstruct breasts after mastectomies. The only research published on the subject up to that time had been ours, so we did not have any outside information to guide us. Our chief problem was capsular contracture, which was much more visible when no real breast was present to help hide it.

I read the study on polyurethane implants and called the inventor-peddler, who came to see me. He told me that everything was true. I called the doctor-promoter, who confirmed this, and because he seemed honest I decided to try them. I can only attribute my naiveté to my youthful inexperience at the time. Perhaps that is why a person two months out of training should not be made chief of services.

In any event, I implanted more than 250 of these prostheses over a one-year period. Fairly soon, though, I found that within days after surgery about ten percent of the patients developed a fiery, red rash and severe itching that lasted about two weeks. In my opinion, this was clearly allergic as it was alleviated by a cortisone-type ointment and an antihistamine pill. I called the "promoter" and the "peddler," but they said they had never seen this reaction and suggested that I must be washing the implants in some strange soap. For months, I spied on the operating room nurses to catch them soaping the implants. They never did.

The fact that some patients had reactions made me uneasy, but the implants did stay miraculously soft at first. However, after about six to eight months, the roof fell in. The implants all started to harden, and the hardening was much worse than with the simple gel-filled implants. The patients started to fill the office. They were almost lined up at the door. I had to hide them from my other patients.

What had happened was that, although the scar tissue fibers that were laid down in the beginning were indeed trapped by the polyurethane, those laid down later were not

The Truth about Breast Implants

in contact with the polyurethane and were not trapped by it. These later layers arranged themselves in parallel rows and did contract. By this time, a considerable amount of scar tissue had already been laid down and mixed with the polyurethane fibers so that the overall capsules were much thicker than even the thickest of the ones we had ever seen before.

Then the worst happened. The polyurethane fibers pulled loose from the implant as the capsule shrank. The result was a shrunken, very hard, totally misshapen implant with major wrinkles where the implant was actually folded over on itself. Bad enough, you might think, but there is more. The implants were not made in one piece and had a weakness where the front and the back were joined. When contracted, they tended to split at this seam and release their silicone gel. It was a nightmare.

Memorial Sloan-Kettering Cancer Center and The New York Hospital (where I also worked) had $10,000 of these implants in inventory when the chicken came home to roost. There was no way, in good conscience, that these could be used. We tossed them all in the garbage, and I apologetically told everybody I knew that they were awful and widely published that opinion. The inventor hasn't spoken to me again to this day. I have removed almost all of these implants from my patients and replaced them with saline-filled ones.

Then, in 1983, my ear perked up in the middle of a national medical conference when I heard the word "polyurethane." I suddenly realized that the speaker was talking about polyurethane-covered breast implants. He said that he had discovered the cure for capsular contracture and that he had used a large number of them for years without any trouble. I found the speaker afterward and mentioned my experience. He said that he was using a new form of polyurethane that didn't have the old problems. I didn't know what to make of it.

Over the next two years, I found that the implants—which had a new name, "Même®"—were being touted by another doctor-promoter, a role I had barely escaped. Over the next few years, large numbers of these implants came to be used. As some of these unfortunate patients found my office, I discovered that they had had the same early allergic disasters and had developed the same delayed tight capsule formation. Their implants had to be removed—a choice many are glad they made now that it also turns out that the breakdown of polyurethane produced TDA (2-toluene diamine), a chemical compound that has caused liver cancer in laboratory animals. In 1991, the FDA began investigating the implants, and newspapers began raising questions about their safety. Soon after, the manufacturer of the Même and Replicon—another foam-covered implant—voluntarily withdrew them from the market, at least until they could do further studies. But plastic surgeons had been debating the carcinogenicity of polyurethane-covered implants for well over ten years before the FDA started sniffing around, and it's doubtful that very many women who got them were informed of the risks.

My Conversion to Saline

By the end of 1978, I decided to use saline implants exclusively. This was not only because they did not leach liquid silicone (and had no polyurethane) but also because the results with saline implants were superior. They looked better from every point of view and stayed softer in much higher numbers, and there was a lower incidence of tight, painful scar tissue formation. Fifteen years and more than two thousand implants later, I am still convinced that saline implants give the best results.

The Revelations

Many Americans were shocked by the revelations about silicone gel–filled breast implants during the FDA hearings that ended in February 1992. Women came forward with severe problems that were at least circumstantially linked with silicone gel–filled implants. Many had what has come to be called "silicone-induced human adjuvant disease," an immune disorder characterized by arthritis, joint pain, skin lesions, malaise, and weight loss. Many also had other medical complaints that were never before associated with breast implants, at least not in the medical literature. Many people wondered how the FDA could allow a substance to be implanted in over two million women for 30 years when it wasn't proven safe. The reason is that silicone gel–filled implants— and breast implants of any kid for that matter—were not subject to approval by the FDA, which had no regulatory authority over implants at all until 1976.

At that time, nearly 15 years after silicone implants were first used, Congress passed a law requiring that new medical devices, meaning anything that was not a drug, be proved safe and effective. Breast implants and all other medical devices already on the market were allowed to stay on the market; they were "grandfathered" in. However, the law did permit the FDA to require manufacturers to provide safety information if questions should arise.

Few plastic surgeons foresaw the backlash, though surely more doctors should have. As far back as 1982, unbeknownst to the public, there were plenty of doubts being raised in the medical journals about silicone gel's safety—enough to raise some eyebrows at the FDA. At that time the agency declared that implants presented a "potential, unreasonable risk of injury" and proposed requiring implant manufacturers to carry out safety and efficacy studies. But the wheels at the FDA grind slowly. It was not until after congressional hearings on implants that the FDA made the regulation final. In July 1991, the new head of the FDA, David Kessler (arguably the most consumer-minded FDA chief to come along), declared that to continue selling their devices, implant makers had to submit marketing applications that included results of safety and efficacy studies they've done.

An FDA advisory panel went over the results of the manufacturers' studies in November 1991. At about that time, juries started making some very large monetary awards to women who sued makers of silicone gel–filled implants, claiming that they were the source of their medical problems. So many questions still remained about silicone gel's safety that, in January 1992, Kessler called for a temporary ban on silicone gel breast implants and for more hearings. Newspapers were filled with stories of memos from Dow Corning staff citing worrisome findings about animal studies with silicone gel. Others suggested that tests with laboratory dogs were purported to show no ill effects of silicone gel when, in fact, one of the dogs used in the experiments died, though Dow

Corning contends that there was no connection. Recently, Dow Corning admitted that some of its inspectors falsified quality control tests of implants before sale. The FDA had even warned Dow Corning in 1991 against misleading women about the safety of silicone gel breast implants in its toll-free telephone hotline.

The FDA Clampdown

On April 16, 1992, the FDA commissioner ruled that so many questions remained about breast implants filled with silicone gel that they would henceforth be available only through controlled clinical studies, results of which would help answer those questions. Kessler explained in a special report in the *New England Journal of Medicine* that it is not known, for instance, how long silicone gel–filled implants last or what percentage rupture. What's more, the chemical composition of the gel that leaks into the body when a breast implant ruptures is unknown. And the link between these implants and immune-related disorders and other systemic diseases is also unclear. Serious questions remain about the ability of manufacturers to produce the device reliably and under strict quality controls. Until these questions are answered, Kessler said, the FDA cannot legally approve the general use of breast implants filled with silicone gel. He dismissed the notion that women ought to be able to decide on their own whether to take the risks associated with silicone gel implants as an "unrealistic burden" on people.

As a result of Kessler's ruling, silicone gel–filled implants were, at first, made available only to women whose need was "urgent," such as those who were already under-going breast reconstruction following cancer surgery. In the next phase, the FDA would allow silicone gel implants to be used only if women agreed to participate in controlled clin-ical studies, meaning that researchers would follow them for many years and record any implant-related problems that arose. In the first study, for instance, silicone gel breast implants would be allowed in some 3,000 women after breast cancer surgery or to correct severe breast deformities or as replacements. The five-year study is aimed at finding the rate of rupture, infection, and contracture. In the last stage, the FDA would permit implants for breast reconstruction or aug-mentation only to a limited number of women who agreed to even more carefully controlled clinical trials.

Awaiting Answers

Until answers are forthcoming, anyone who gets silicone gel–filled implants is simply challenging fate. As a spokes-man for the national Y-Me breast cancer information and support organization said in congressional hearings last April, "Each new ache, pain, or itch is self-analyzed with silicone foremost under consideration as the culprit." If liquid silicone is responsible for scleroderma or rheumatoid arthritis or any of the other diseases with which it is being connected, it's particularly bad because those diseases are painful, disfiguring, and even crippling. The plastic surgery community right now should be saying, "We regret that we ever used these implants. We hope and pray that they are not responsible for any of the symptoms that people have claimed. Though we saw suggestive studies, we never dreamed that this was a possibility. We're pigheaded. But at least now we have made a determination that we are not going to use silicone gel–filled implants any more—or at least until we can be sure that they are not harmful." But, unfortunately, the reaction of the vast majority of plastic surgeons is far from this. Most are not being so open, and most have still not accepted that they should stop using gel-filled implants until they are proved safe. Amazingly, most plastic surgeons think that someone should have to prove them unsafe before they should have to stop using them.

The War Chest

You'd think that plastic surgeons would just forget about silicone gel–filled implants and start using the saline implants. I suppose they're afraid that they will make it easier for patients to sue or to win suits if they give in. And it seems that plastic surgeons will keep fighting for silicone gel–filled implants. In the fall of 1991, the American Society of Plastic and Reconstructive Surgeons (ASPRS), the professional umbrella organization, began assessing each of its 5,000 members $1,050 over a three-year period to fund a party-line response to "critical public policy issues." The society's latest invoice warns doctors who refuse to support its efforts by not paying up that their "membership will be terminated." So far, about $2.7 million has been collected. According to the society, about $1 million has been spent on national lobbying and "individual members' government efforts."

The Quest for Perfect Breasts

I'm sure the society thinks its war chest is money well spent. The ASPRS even gloats that high-level conversations between its representatives and the FDA won the elimination of discussion about the possibility of untoward effects of silicone gel–filled implants on breast feeding and birth defects in patient information documents. "In what is one of ASPRS' greatest victories in the breast controversy to date," says the society's September 1992 *Special Bulletin*, "the FDA has agreed to revise its mandatory informed consent document . . . to reflect changes proposed by the Society." According to the official newsletter, those changes included deleting a statement that silicone gel–filled breast implants can cause problems with breast feeding and deleting negative statements about the procedure of breaking up implant capsules through manual pressure. The newsletter notes that those deletions were "especially important because the original wording exposed physicians who chose to perform the procedure to possible litigation."

If there is evidence that babies breastfed by women with silicone gel–filled implants are taking in silicone in droplet form, can anybody say that this is not harmful? It seems to me that the burden of proof is on the surgeon and manufacturers to prove that these implants and the liquid silicone traveling in the body and traveling to a baby are not harmful. If they can't prove that, they've got no business marketing or implanting them. What are they going to say if 20 years from now it's absolutely proved that this caused damage? They'll say how sorry they were and that they didn't know better, and they're going to be exactly in the same posture as the cigarette companies and salesmen. I find this attitude impossible to defend, even obnoxious.

Scrutinizing Saline

Although Kessler has said that saline-filled implants are far less worrisome because they are filled with sterile salt-water instead of silicone gel, he promised that saline-filled implants would get a full review. Saline-filled implants, after all, do have an outer shell of solid silicone. If it had been up to me, I would have held hearings on saline-filled implants even before silicone gel–filled implants. I understand that Kessler went after silicone gel–filled implants because, from a public health point of view, they pose the most potential risk.

But my suspicion is that when saline-filled implants are determined to be safe, it will be realized that someone foresaw an immense public outcry if it was revealed that plastic surgeons had deliberately chosen not to use them for 15 years. Reviewing saline-filled implants first might have shown women that at least there was something available that was proven safe that they could use. (For details, see Chapter 5.) Instead, over a year of public worry has been very unintelligently created by the FDA, well-meaning or not.

New Types of Breast Implants

Naturally, some investigators are busy experimenting with new substances for filling implants. But remember our inventor-peddler and doctor-promoter characters. In my middle age, I've found that it is a very good idea to maintain a healthy skepticism about anything new that comes along, considering what's been tried in the past. Most often, a doctor-promoter redesigns an implant slightly and touts it as a breakthrough, reporting on it at medical conferences and in journals, and a company or inventor peddles it afterward. The "invented here" syndrome leads to many serious presentations before national conventions that simply don't pan out.

Until I see more studies that are scientifically valid, for instance, I will remain skeptical about the efforts underway at Washington University School of Medicine in St. Louis, where researchers are developing peanut-oil implants. "Peanut oil filled implants are nontoxic, biodegradable and absorbable," says V. Leroy Young, a professor of plastic and reconstructive surgery who is involved in the effort. "If for some reason they would leak, the oil would simply be absorbed by the body."

Although the St. Louis team has published a number of studies on peanut oil's potential use in implants, one must be very skeptical that peanut oil will not cause very severe body reactions. For instance, it is one of the worst irritants to the lungs; peanut oil from an inhaled nut, for instance, often induces pneumonia that is frequently fatal. So why would anyone deliberately put it into the breast? Another advantage, they say, is that under laboratory conditions breast X rays pass through peanut oil, yielding unobscured mammograms, which are so important for picking up tiny tumors when they are most treatable. Silicone gel heavily obscures breast X rays and saline less so, as I'll discuss in Chapter 6. But the idea that peanut oil is more translucent than simple saline seems odd on the basis of early impressions. We have been burned too many times. The burden of truth must be on the claimer.

The so-called MISTI GOLD™ implants filled with Bio-Oncotic™ gel were marketed for awhile on the basis that they didn't interfere as much with mammograms and that they were "biocompatible," which implies that they simulate normal body tissues—thus, no reaction, no scar tissue, no tight capsule. The maker, BioPlasty of St. Paul, Minnesota, said that instead of silicone gel, the implant was comprised mostly of a polymer gel called "plasdone Au24K." It was claimed that the MISTI GOLD stayed softer longer. But when the FDA started questioning some of the claims and asking for information about the filling, the implants went off the market in the U.S.

There have been implants made that have lateral extensions on them to try to fill the area under the arm where fat and lymph nodes are removed after cancer surgery. There are also oddly shaped add-on implants that you can insert next to the main implant to fill out hollows. Neither of these ideas has been successful.

Even when false claims are not purposely made, the rule rather than the exception is that articles that are written early are full of claims and hope. Doctors are rarely as quick to submit articles or deliver subsequent papers if, as happens in the majority of cases, the concept later turns out not to be as good as was originally thought. Yet, as Chapter 4 shows, doctors have reported problems that arose with silicone gel–filled implants over the past 30 years. As you'll see, many of those reports had a shocking chauvinistic "among us" tone to them and were definitely not meant to be read by the general public.

2

〜

Making Informed Choices

**Preparing to See
Your Doctor**

Young and older women alike choose to undergo breast reconstruction after cancer surgery, or mastectomy, because they want to look their best and feel comfortable. They want to feel free engaging in physical activity. They want to go to cocktail parties and wear something low-cut again. At first, it might seem that younger women would have a harder time coping with a mastectomy and the reconstruction process, but many seem able to deal with it more easily. I can remember two women in their early 20s who had cancer and sailed through their reconstruction effortlessly with a "this is unpleasant but let's get it over with" attitude. Their mothers, on the other hand, did most of the worrying and were guilt-ridden that somehow they had passed on the "bad" gene that made this happen to their daughters.

As for women who come in not for reconstruction but for enlargement of small breasts, implants promise an end to what may seem like a torturous source of disappointment. It goes without saying that implants do not automatically solve life's problems. A small-breasted young woman may feel that if she only had large breasts she wouldn't be sitting home without a date. I've seen many single women who thought they'd get married if only they had larger breasts. Such women will likely be disappointed. There may be any number of reasons a woman is not in a relationship, but very small breasted women often fixate on their breast size. The psychological benefits for most women are extraordinarily good. I have seen young women absolutely blossom just because they have the reinforcement of having larger breasts; they start to smile. They become more popular not because they have bigger breasts but because they gain self-confidence. This chapter will help set the record straight about available options so that women can make informed choices and find the help they need.

Breast Reconstruction after Mastectomy

Many women considering breast reconstruction confided to my longtime nurse, Irene Landry, that they no longer let their husbands see them naked. They would wear their bra and prosthesis—an artificial breast form worn in the bra—even when making love. Many never wore V-necked blouses or shirts, fearing that someone would notice the prosthesis or, worse yet, that the prosthesis might pop out. For these women, the psychological scars of mastectomy never healed.

When they looked down while in the shower, they were always reminded of the cancer and of their loss.

So many times, concerned husbands would pull Irene aside at the office and plead with her to convince their wives that they still loved them, that they still found them attractive. Many were worried that their wives were considering reconstruction not for themselves but for their mates. "Irene, talk to her; tell her she shouldn't do this for me," one man said. "She isn't doing this for you," Irene would reply matter-of-factly. "She is doing this for herself." No amount of flattery could convince these women that they still looked attractive. They had to feel it themselves. Breast reconstruction does not change everything about life after mastectomy. It will not ease the effects of chemotherapy or dispel worries about recurrence. But it will instantly give women back a very good semblance of their natural appearance and wipe away a radically altered self-image.

A Permanent Solution

Breast reconstruction is a permanent solution; for most women, a prosthesis is not. That's especially true for large-breasted women who need a big prosthesis to look natural. Prostheses are heavy and feel hot in the summer. They hang heavily on the shoulder and have an uncanny propensity to pop out of bathing suits and tennis outfits. The woman must wear her bra at all times to look and feel "normal." Otherwise, she feels off balance.

To approximate the feeling, take your right hand and place it on your left shoulder. Now, get up and try to walk a straight line. Feels strange, doesn't it? This off-centered feeling is only part of what a woman who's lost a breast has to deal with.

I have quite a few patients who are in their sixties or older. Some are a little sheepish at first, fearing that Irene and I would think them foolish for choosing reconstruction at their age. They quickly get over this feeling, though, after discovering that their bodies can be virtually restored to the way they were before their mastectomies.

Some patients decide to augment their other, healthy breast at the time of reconstruction if they feel that they want to be larger anyway. Often, unless that's done, women whose breasts were very small to begin with may look a little lopsided after reconstruction. But I recall a number of patients who I really thought should have had their normal breasts made larger to match, though they were adamant about leaving them alone. I reconstructed only their surgically removed sides using very small implants, and, though their breasts didn't match as well as they might have, they were quite happy with the results.

Immediate Reconstruction

Ostensibly to spare women discomfort, many breast surgeons today offer their mastectomy patients the option of immediate breast reconstruction with a temporary expander implant placed under the chest muscles right after the breast is removed. During weekly office visits, the temporary implant is expanded little by little with weekly injections of saline through the skin into a special type of valve that will not leak.

Making Informed Choices

As the implant expands, it stretches the chest skin so that after three months a pocket has formed that is large enough to hold a permanent implant. During a second surgery, then, the temporary expander implant is removed, and a permanent implant is inserted.

Though immediate reconstruction sounds like a good idea, a large number unfortunately turn out poorly because of complications. For instance, the risk of infection following mastectomy is greater if an expander implant is used immediately. And the recuperation period is longer and more painful. What's more, it's far more common for the implant to end up in the wrong position after immediate reconstruction because the muscle attachments are in the way and cannot be released. But if you wait about three months, you can avoid all the pain and problems that go hand in hand with temporary expander implants by simply inserting a permanent saline-filled implant. Until this pernicious idea of immediate reconstruction came among us, I reconstructed everyone two to three months later with no trouble.

Despite this, I find myself in the position of having to do immediate reconstructions because of the pressures from surgeons and patients. In fact, immediate reconstruction benefits everyone but the patient. Breast surgeons may tell patients it's best, but really they prefer immediate reconstruction because they can leave the operating room as soon as the breast is removed, leaving the plastic surgeon to stop the bleeding and close the wound. The plastic surgeon also takes on most of the postoperative care. The work of the breast surgeon is cut in half.

Many plastic surgeons are eager to do immediate reconstruction because they get the patient not through their competence but because of a relationship with the breast surgeon. The patient does not get a chance to research the credentials of the plastic surgeon, who, as often as not, knows little about breast reconstruction. The truth is that the relationship between the breast surgeon and the plastic surgeon is usually not due to professional respect (which the breast surgeon is not usually competent to judge anyway) but more often because they are partners at the tennis club or their wives are friends or their children play on the same Little League team. Perhaps now that this little secret is out, this operating room charade of pushing for immediate reconstruction will finally let up.

Breast Augmentation

Most of the women who seek breast enlargement or augmentation are truly small-breasted. They suffer embarrassment about their size, especially when dressed in summer wear and bathing suits (which are particularly difficult for small-breasted women to find in the right size) as well as during intimate situations. On the whole, small-breasted women don't want to be large-breasted sex bombs; they just want to look "normal" and to be able to buy clothing easily. A smaller number seek breast enlargement after a large weight loss or when they're through breast feeding, after which it's common for breasts to lose volume and look droopy. For these women, implants can often provide a better look, although in some situations a breast lift by excising and tightening excess skin is warranted. The latter leads to extensive, visible scarring and should not be undertaken lightly.

It's rare that a woman isn't a good candidate for augmentation. That's true whether a woman has small breasts (or even no breasts at all) or whether she has a chest wall that is fairly flat in the front or that comes to a point at the sternum like the bow of a ship. Women with both body types can attain the shape they seek using implants. Even a history of cancer in the family or of multiple biopsies for lumps does not mean a woman is not a good candidate for augmentation. Because the implant is placed behind the breast tissue, the breasts can still be examined.

Finding a Surgeon

Finding a surgeon who is truly knowledgeable about breast augmentation and reconstruction won't be easy. Not surprisingly, the least reliable way is to read an advertisement that says that Dr. X can make you look like the 21-year-old model or starlet pictured. Reputable physicians do not advertise. Unfortunately, even asking your own internist, family physician, gynecologist, or even a breast surgeon may not be of much help. Medicine has become so specialized, so compartmentalized, that other physicians know practically nothing about plastic surgery. Again, as likely as not, the plastic surgeon your doctor recommends is a golf partner.

One good strategy, however, is to seek out a plastic surgeon who is on the faculty of the closest medical school. Those will be among the top physicians in your area. That's because academic rank in a medical school is the most difficult credential to earn. In fact, it's a red flag if a plastic surgeon practices in the neighborhood of a medical school and yet is not on the faculty. What's more, the higher their rank, the better; it means that they have been considered best by their colleagues or peers. A full clinical professor is higher than an associate professor, for instance. Any rank of professor is superior to an instructor or someone without academic rank at all. Because breast reconstruction is much more complicated than a simple cosmetic implantation, women who are having a breast rebuilt, even months or years after a mastectomy, would do especially well to look to the expertise available at a major medical center.

For women who seek a plastic surgeon for cosmetic augmentation, the best recommendation will come from someone you know (or a friend of a friend) who has had it done successfully. Of course, one swallow doesn't make a summer; it would be better if you knew several people who had good experiences.

What to Ask

Once you find your way to a plastic surgeon who does breast implantation, you'll need to know what to ask. Following are a dozen questions to consider asking your prospective plastic surgeon for both augmentation and reconstruction. Because this is an emotional meeting for most women, it's a good idea to bring along a notepad to jot down your doctor's answers. Otherwise, many women leave, only to realize later that they had been so unsettled they couldn't remember anything the doctor had said. It is normal to be billed for the initial visit; advice from an expert is valuable. It is perfectly fine for women to see only one surgeon, provided they have done the checks mentioned above.

Making Informed Choices

1. *Are you certified by the American Board of Plastic Surgery?* You can check by calling the American Board of Medical Specialties (ABMS), the oversight organization for board certification, at (800) 776-2378. There are many phoney boards that are more like private clubs, with minimal or no requirements for membership in terms of education and experience, that are not recognized by the ABMS.

2. *What percentage of your practice is devoted to breast augmentation or reconstruction?* Though plastic surgeons typically do many types of procedures, you may want to pick a doctor who specializes in the type of surgery you are looking for. If the surgeon says he does only breasts or, at least, specializes in breast surgery, telephone later using a different name and ask the same questions about a face lift. If the surgeon or his office say that he or she specializes in face lifts, you know whom to stay away from.

3. *What type of augmentation or reconstructive procedure is appropriate for me and why?* Women in search of a better cosmetic look will want to find out if enlargement with implants is best or whether a breast "lift" is what's called for. For some women who've had a mastectomy, breast reconstruction using a flap of muscle tissue from the back, abdomen, or buttock is a viable, though far riskier, option than implants. I'll tell you about that option in Chapter 3.

4. *What type of implant is best?* Of course, I feel quite strongly that saline-filled implants are the best for women who want breast enlargement as well as for those who require breast reconstruction. Specifically, I have had the best results with a round, low-profile, smooth-walled

The Truth about Breast Implants

implant with a positive self-sealing valve. I'll explain what that means in Chapter 5.

5. *Where do you prefer making the incision for implant insertion?* The incision can be made around the nipple, in the armpit, or at the fold under the breast. I prefer the latter because that approach best ensures proper placement of the implant behind the breast, has the least chance of reducing nipple sensation, and leaves the least noticeable scar.

6. (For mastectomy patients) *Can we achieve a match without augmenting or reducing the size of my natural breast?* The main concern may be simply to ensure that the breasts match well enough for a proper fit in a bra. However, very small breasted women may wish to consider augmentation of the healthy breast; women with very large breasts might wish to inquire about matching the new breast with a smaller natural one through breast-reduction surgery.

7. (For mastectomy patients) *If transplanted tissue is used, where do you suggest it come from? Will I require an implant as well?* As you'll learn later in this chapter and in more detail in Chapter 3, transplanted tissue can come from the back, abdomen, or buttock. But an implant may still be necessary to give the projection needed for a natural-looking breast.

8. *Will I be able to wear revealing clothes?* Enlargement procedures obviously demand that breasts look and feel natural in and out of clothes; reconstruction should enable women's breasts to look natural when wearing bras, bathing suits, and strapless dresses.

9. *If after cosmetic enlargement I decide that I really want to be larger or smaller, will you charge for the further surgery?* Because it

Making Informed Choices

really is impossible to know how you're going to like the way your breasts look without actually seeing for yourself after the swelling has gone down a few weeks after surgery, I tell my patients that, if they decide later to be larger or smaller, I'll change the implants free of charge, though they will have to pay any hospital or anesthesia not covered by insurance. (It is usually covered.) I think that women should expect that of any reputable doctor.

10. *If touch-up procedures such as repositioning the implant are necessary, is that covered by your basic surgical fee?* It should be. The standard practice is that there is no charge to the patient by the doctor. As in the answer above, patients will have to pay any hospital costs, though it's usually covered by insurance.

11. *May I see before-and-after photos of actual procedures, including the flap donor sites?* You should expect doctors to show actual, untouched-up photos of their patients from the neck down.

12. *May I speak to any of your patients who have had breast reconstruction or enlargement?* Doctors should be expected to try to put you in touch with several patients who've consented to help out in this way, though it is, of course, unlikely that a doctor would pick anyone who had an unsatisfactory result. In fairness, it must also be said that, although patients who have had their breasts reconstructed after a mastectomy are usually happy to "show and tell," cosmetic enlargement patients are much less ready to do so.

At follow-up visits, you'll want to discuss in detail the type of procedure the doctor thinks is best. There are two major types of operations: those that use implants and those that use the patient's own tissues. As you'll see, implantation is a relatively simple procedure, and transplantation is quite complex. On the following pages, I'll map out the major steps of both types of procedures just to give you an idea of what's involved.

What to Expect during Cosmetic Enlargement

Your doctor will likely start off by showing you a book of pictures of previous patients who have undergone cosmetic breast enlargement surgery. In my practice, some are as small as an A cup and some a middle B, large B, small C, big C, and D. I ask, "Of all of these, which one looks the best to you?" At first, the patients are always a little embarrassed and reluctant to pick a large size. And sometimes they're a little undecided, but we start to get an idea. And then I ask the patient to go out and buy some Victoria's Secret catalogs or *Playboy* magazines and find pictures that show breasts that look best to them and to bring them to the office.

The photos give me a very good idea about what size they want to be. Obviously, if a woman wants to be too big and it's unrealistic, I'll tell her that I don't think it's a very good idea. Besides looking odd, inappropriately large implants can cause a woman to develop furrowing of the shoulders from the weight of wearing a bra. Exercise would be uncomfortable; the breasts might even get in the way. Later in life, she would risk painful sagging. In the end, we settle on a size that's right and then schedule a time for surgery. Before the malpractice rates and problems became so onerous, I used to perform cosmetic enlargements in the office. It is no longer worth the cost and hassles because of the requirements of government and insurance companies. In addition, most hospitals have now developed good same-day surgery facilities, which is where I now perform cosmetic enlargement. Of course, reconstruction after mastectomy requires an overnight stay, and I have always done this in the hospital.

When the day of the operation arrives, I sit the patient on the operating room table and take some "before" pictures so that she can compare the result objectively a few weeks later. Because most women don't carry their shoulders level, I often have to coax them into straightening their shoulders properly. That's important to ensure that the bottom of the two breasts are at the same level. Then I actually draw a mark at the underside of each breast right in the fold, or "infra-mammary crease." This ensures that the two breasts will match after the implants are in place. I then take the magazine pictures that they have given me and tape them up around the walls of the operating room so that the surgical team understands the end result that we're after.

I ask the patient to lie down, and another doctor, an anesthesiologist, either puts her to sleep using general anesthesia or we use a combination of heavy sedation and novocaine. Then I draw a circle 16 centimeters in diameter on the chest around the nipple. That mark helps me place the implant into a pocket centered directly behind the nipple. That's important because if the implant is inserted off the mark, the nipple would look too high, too low, or off center. It also helps me match the breasts' bottom creases. In some women, the nipples are not at the same height on the chest.

In such cases, a compromise must be made so that there are only slight differences between the position of the nipples and the bottoms of the breasts. Fortunately, this is rare, but when it exists it is essential to spot it in advance.

When everything is mapped out, the patient is prepped with iodine and draped with sterile towels. I make an inch- or inch-and-a-half-long incision, which will be virtually undetectable because it is tucked up under the breast in the bottom crease and off to the side a little. I separate the backside of the breast tissue from the front side of the muscle, which is like opening a piece of pita bread, until I open a space out to the periphery of those markings.

Some doctors are now promoting the idea that if the implant is behind the muscle, one can get a better mammogram, or breast X ray, because the thickness of the muscle is between the implant and the breast tissue. Many doctors have sold that to an awful lot of people, but it's absolute nonsense. The muscle is so thin that getting a three-sixteenths-inch advantage doesn't do very much to separate the breast from the implant. In my opinion, the muscle, when in front of the implant, can even obscure mammograms by casting its own shadow.

For cosmetic augmentation, I never make the pocket behind the muscle. With breast tissue and normal skin and fat in front of the implant, there's no reason to do that. Putting an implant in behind the muscle certainly doesn't solve the problem of painful hardening of the implant—what is called "capsular contracture." The muscle layer is supposed to hide it somewhat, but it does not do this effectively. The steps that most prevent capsular contracture are simply good sterile technique, keeping bleeding to a minimum, and using saline implants. Perhaps the principle reason to avoid going under the muscle in cosmetic augmentation is that disturbing the area between the muscle and ribs frequently causes scar tissue to develop. If scar tissue does form and binds the muscle and the implant to the ribs, the result is usually permanent soreness and a limitation of arm motion.

After the pocket is made, I use a sizer implant, which comes in increments of thirty cubic centimeters, which equals one ounce. Sizer implants are much thicker walled than a permanent implant and can be sterilized and reused. I fill the sizer with what I estimate to be the right amount of saline and place it in the pocket behind the breast as a trial. Then I stop and look. This part of the surgery is very much an art. Sometimes implants that you thought would be perfect make the breasts look funny. They look too round, project too much, look stretched, or just look too big. At this point, the surgeon's aesthetic sense is paramount to how pleasing the final appearance is. If the implant looks too large or small, then I go to the next sizer implant down or up. When I've found the best size for the look the patient is after, I take out the sizer and replace it with a permanent implant, which I fill with saline. I usually add a very small amount of cortisone, which leaches out of the implant over the following six weeks and tends to keep scar tissue from forming tight bonds.

Patients can't be expected to make the final decision about the size of the implants because they are sedated, if not asleep, and really couldn't see very well anyway. Even so, I know that some of my colleagues sit up their patients and say, "Take a look. This is your last chance." They do this so that if a patient comes back in two months and says she'd like to be bigger, they can try to charge them all over again. "You made your decision," those doctors will say, "now, it's not my problem." Well, that's unreasonable, in my opinion.

Occasionally, implants of different sizes have to be used on the two sides because breasts themselves are not always the same size. Patients accept that from Mother Nature, but I can assure you that they do not accept it from a surgeon at the end of such an operation. When we're finished, I close the incision, leaving drainage tubes in overnight to suck out any blood that pools. Finally, I wrap the patient's chest in elastic bandages to provide some compression, which reduces the chance of bleeding in the pocket.

The next day, when I ask her to sit up so I can check the incisions, she'll get her first peek at her new breasts and sometimes say, "Oh, no! Those are too big." And I say, "Live with them for a few weeks while the swelling goes down." I know that, for most women, their self-image will change. When they first go out, they feel as if their breasts are sticking out and so they hunch over. Some put overcoats on when they go to the market because they're afraid that, if they don't, the grocery boys will follow them down the street. After awhile, of course, they find that they really like the way they look. Only about 1 in 20 patients wants to be larger; I can't remember the last time anybody wanted to be smaller.

What to Expect during Breast Reconstruction

The procedure for putting in the implant for reconstruction following mastectomy—removal of the breast tissue—is very similar to the one for breast enlargement. First, before surgery, I ask the patient to sit up, make sure her shoulders are straight, and take some "before" pictures.

Then I draw a mark in the crease underneath the remaining breast. Using a level ruler, I draw a line on the mastectomy side that will serve as the incision point, and I also determine the bottom crease of the new breast. A woman who has had both breasts removed needs to bring a bra with her to the operating room. She puts artificial prostheses in the bra cups and adjusts the straps so that the breasts are in the position on her chest that her original breasts were in (the position that fits her clothes). The bottom of the bra cups determines the bottom of the new breasts. I make sure that the marks are level, and then I draw a circular dotted line on the chest that's usually about 14 to 15 centimeters in diameter to represent the position of the new breast. Then, as with women undergoing augmentation, the patient lies down, and another doctor administers anesthesia. (General anesthesia is always used for breast reconstruction, but later, if nipple reconstruction is attempted, local anesthesia is often all that is needed.)

After she is prepped, I make the incision through the skin and the fat until the underlying muscle is exposed. Although most of the breast tissue has been removed, it is sometimes still possible to make a pocket for the implant over the muscle. The closer the implant is to the skin, by and large, the better it looks, but the more risk there is of it eventually wearing through the skin. That's because after a mastectomy, skin that's stretched over the chest is thin and has a very limited blood supply. On the other hand, the muscle has a very good blood supply. It's almost impossible for implants behind the muscle to extrude through the skin.

The Truth about Breast Implants

In optimal cases, I can split the muscle. That strategy doesn't affect the muscle strength afterward and doesn't risk violating the sliding plane (the area where the muscle slides on the chest wall), so there's far less risk that the chest will hurt or feel tight or that arm movement will be affected.

As in cosmetic augmentation, the pocket for the implant is made by separating the muscle or fat at the appropriate level, as I've said, like opening a piece of pita bread. Once a pocket of the proper size for the implant has been formed and any bleeding has been stopped, the implant is filled with saline and is put in through the incision. If its size, looseness, and position are correct, the incision is closed. As in simple augmentation, a suction drain is left in overnight because there's always a bit of weeping and pooling of blood after the surgery, and you don't want blood to cake around the implant. Blood clots and makes the implants feel hard. Finally, elastic bandages are put on the chest in a crisscross, soldier boy fashion to put a little pressure on the chest and help prevent bleeding.

The next morning the drains come out, and the dressing is changed. I tell patients to try to keep the bandages on for about a week, but if they become desperate, usually due to itching, they can take them off after three or four days. After a week, I take the stitches out.

At that point, they can put on a bra and lead a fairly unrestricted, normal life. They still can't do anything strenuous, such as tennis, golf, jogging, or exercise class, for about three weeks after surgery. But they can do normal things right away, like drive a car, go for long walks, push a cart in a market, or reach up into shelves.

The shape of the final result is not totally controllable by the plastic surgeon. As long as the surgery was done correctly, it is gravity and the way the skin stretches that determine the shape of the breast over the subsequent six to eight weeks. I joke with my patients that we are all in the hands of God and we all know how difficult She can be.

Tissue Transfer Procedures: Are They Worth It?

Transplanting muscle, fat, and skin tissue from the back, abdomen, or buttock to the breast is offered as a way to avoid the problems of implants altogether. But tissue transfer operations are major procedures, and they are also by far the riskiest options in breast reconstruction. I am among a growing number of doctors who believe that the desire of some plastic surgeons to prove that they can move tissue from anywhere in the body to the breast has overcome good sense and good taste.

The most complicated and most dangerous tissue transfer procedure, the TRAM flap (so named in 1982 for transverse rectus abdominus myocutaneous), requires a flap of transferred abdominal rectus muscle from the stomach area. The island of skin, fat, and muscle tissue from the belly is cut out in such a way that it's kept connected to its main blood supply. Next, an opening is made under the skin of the mastectomized area to accommodate the transplanted belly tissue. A tunnel is created under the skin from the abdomen to the breast, and the flap is carefully pushed through that tunnel and popped into the breast area, where it is shaped and sewn in place. The stomach is given a type of tummy tuck. Later, a nipple can be grafted on to the reconstructed breast to complete the effect.

The Truth about Breast Implants

When successful, the transplant can result in a very pleasing, soft contour that looks quite natural in a bra. But the downside risks are so severe that, in my view, they would be acceptable only if the patient's life were at stake. To me, these risks are totally unacceptable when they are borne just to give someone a new breast. Patients who have lost a breast are usually in a fragile state. They are not always thinking clearly, and they are largely dependent on what their doctors tell them. If the doctor says he can create a new breast that is natural (not an implant) using their own tissues, most patients eagerly agree. When the offer also promises a flatter tummy, it's almost more than a woman with a poor body image can resist.

It's so appealing that it seems too good to be true. And in my opinion it is just that. Not only have there been deaths from this procedure, but the risk is high that the tissue transfer will not take. Physicians are finding that in ten percent of cases, some or all of the transplanted tissue dies within a few days because of an insufficient blood supply. If some of the breast tissue dies, the only way to repair the damage is with—what else?—an implant. Even when the transplant takes, the incidence of lower abdominal hernias that are hard to fix is alarmingly high. And the final blow is that the promised tummy tuck usually fails, resulting in a waistline that is paradoxically larger than before because of the way the stomach tends to bulge over the scar line at the sides. Sometimes, you just have to shake your head in wonderment that doctors haven't abandoned the procedure altogether. (More on this in Chapter 3.)

Buttock tissue transfers have many of the same problems as TRAM transfers except that if the flap dies, you will have suffered only a disfigured, occasionally painful buttock instead of a totally screwed up abdomen. In that sense, they are preferable to abdominal tissue transfers, but not by much. The procedure requires a sophisticated microsurgical connection of the transferred blood vessels. If this procedure is not done well, all the transplanted tissue will die. Also, these techniques may take as long as 12 hours to complete. And most surgeons are not highly skilled in microvascular surgery, so the incidence of risks like the development of life-threatening clots or complications from prolonged anesthesia are significant.

Neither the TRAM, the buttock, nor most other tissue transfer procedures make any sense compared to simple implantation. Saline-filled implants take only about 40 minutes to put in and are without any real risk, except that they might get hard, leak, or not be in the right position. But these are extremely minor complications in comparison with those seen in tissue transfers gone bad. And they are easily fixable; failed tissue transfers are not.

The only reasons I can think of that surgeons are eager to do these procedures are that misleading claims about their benefits attract patients—and insurance payments are much higher than for simple implants. I'll discuss these procedures in more detail in the next chapter.

Lumpectomy Questions

It's possible that all breast reconstruction procedures may fall out of use over the coming decade as more women opt for breast-saving lumpectomies instead of mastectomy.

The Truth about Breast Implants

The attraction of lumpectomy, of course, is that although as much as a quarter of the breast may be removed and the breast left smaller, at least it is a woman's own natural breast.

But is lumpectomy really a better cancer operation? The truth is that because the lumpectomy is not yet twenty years old, we don't know for sure what the long-term result is going to be. To comprehend the significance, one needs only remember that in the early 1960s Robert McWhirter of Scotland was one of the prime proponents of doing simple mastectomies for breast cancer: just removing the breast tissue, then irradiating the lymph nodes. His early results in the first ten years were better than even the radical mastectomies that were being done in those days. But in the second ten years the results completely fell apart, and there was a great increase in cancer recurrence. Today we are just getting into the second decade of lumpectomies, and, although radiation is supposed to kill off all the remaining nests of cancerous cells, not enough time has yet passed to know for sure what long-term recurrence rates may be like. I certainly have seen plenty of them in my office. What's more, studies in the medical literature are beginning to suggest that women who've had intensive radiation are starting to show up in doctors' offices with lung damage from the radiation. Women, it seems, still are not being completely informed about the risks.

3

⚬⚭

Transplant Surgery

The Riskiest
Procedures Yield the
Poorest Results

Increasingly, surgeons are selling patients on the idea that they can fashion breasts out of their own body tissues and thus avoid using implants after mastectomy. Though this may be ingenious in theory, the end result is seldom as good as it might be if only a simple saline-filled implant were used. What's more, the procedures for transferring tissue are certainly more complicated and dangerous. Sometimes it seems that surgeons are too interested in confronting the unknown and developing new and risky procedures that they can name after themselves. I suppose that for some restless minds, the everyday, simple, and reliable procedure is just too boring.

Tissue transfers to make a new breast go back to the late 1950s, when the earliest "all-natural" procedure was developed. This was done on large-breasted women on whom doctors attempted to reduce the size of the healthy breast and transplant the leftover tissue to the mastectomized side.

The Truth about Breast Implants

It was tried repeatedly but never worked. The results were always awful.

The latest version of tissue transfers—a major escalation in complexity, risk, and foolishness—is the TRAM flap transfer. Doctors take an expanse of skin, fat, and muscle from the lower belly, move it to the chest, and shape it into a breastlike mound. Surgeons promise that because no artificial implants are used, the operation is better and less risky. In fact, the procedure is the riskiest of all options—some patients have even died from blockages to blood vessels in the lungs as a result of the surgery. In one study of 82 patients who had TRAM flaps, doctors at M. D. Anderson Cancer Center and Baylor College of Medicine reported that about 42 percent of markedly obese patients experienced complications such as infections, deep vein clots, partial loss of flap tissue, or abdominal bulges. Such complications also struck one in three moderately obese patients and one in four average-weight patients. If the FDA is looking for something to outlaw, this is it. Unfortunately, the government has absolutely no say in the matter; it is outside of the FDA's jurisdiction because no medical "device" is involved.

There are, of course, other tissue transfer procedures, including one that I feel is beneficial and many more that lack varying degrees of appeal and justification. None, however, are for women who wish only to enlarge small breasts. The risks are so much greater than simple implantation and the results so many orders of magnitude less pleasing that their use is unthinkable for breast augmentation. Following are some of the other tissue transfer procedures along with their pros and cons.

Back Muscle Transfer (Latissimus Dorsi Muscle Transfer)

This procedure is the one exception to my dislike for tissue transfers. In this operation, doctors transfer a flap of muscle and sometimes skin from a mastectomy patient's back around to her chest. The transferred tissue fills in unsightly hollows left by breast removal surgery and provides a layer of tissue strong enough to hold a saline-filled implant. Later, nipple reconstruction completes the reconstruction (more about nipple reconstruction later in this chapter). It is, of course, important to be sure that the muscle transfer is necessary. I am sorry to say that many of these procedures are being done in people who do not have unsightly hollows and, in fact, have adequate tissue remaining to cover an implant.

To find the back muscle used in this procedure, place both hands on your hips and push downward and backward at the same time. The latissimus dorsi is the large muscle that tightens from the armpit down across the back. In the doctor's office, a woman who is a candidate for this procedure can expect to undergo tests to ensure that the muscle is functioning and has a good blood supply.

On the day of surgery, I sit the patient up and, with a washable marker, draw necessary landmarks on her chest and back, including a line on the mastectomy side that is level with the bottom of the healthy breast. I then outline the area of skin and muscle on the patient's back that will be swung over to the chest. The anesthesiologist then puts the patient to sleep, and she is placed on her side. The back incisions almost completely free the back muscle and skin, leaving it connected to the body only by their blood vessels and nerves. The mastectomy scar in front is opened, and a tunnel is created under the skin through which the transplanted tissue is passed from the back to the front of the chest. If any skin has been brought from the back with the muscle, it is used to relax tight chest skin in front. The transferred muscle is spread out and sewn in place on the chest. A small saline implant is usually placed temporarily under the muscle. (It will be replaced with a larger, properly sized saline implant a few months later after the transferred tissue has healed.) This transfer procedure usually takes about three-and-a-half hours, compared with one hour to place a saline-filled implant.

Though patients usually go home a day or two after surgery, back drains are left in to guard against fluid buildup. They are removed in the doctor's office after a week; the last of the sutures are taken out after two weeks. Strenuous activities such as tennis, golf, and jogging cannot be resumed for three weeks after surgery. Afterward, there is no loss of range of motion in the arm or back, no loss of strength, and no noticeable depression in back from the missing muscle. By and large, when necessary, this is a very good operation with few risks. Though patients are left with a new scar on the back, they are able once again to wear low-cut dresses.

If the back muscle is unusable, say, because doctors have cut the nerve that serves it during the mastectomy, it's time to stop and rethink the whole idea of breast reconstruction. Simple implantation is one thing. Even a latissimus dorsi muscle flap coupled with an implant is a major escalation that patients nonetheless usually consider worth the discomfort and risk. However, the alternative operations discussed below are, in my opinion, dangerous. I would not personally assume the risks, especially considering the poor visual results often attained even when technically successful.

Buttock Transfers

Transplanting a block of tissue from the buttock requires a plastic surgeon skilled in both microsurgery and breast reconstruction. To begin, the doctor injects a small artery that supplies blood to a part of the buttock muscle, or gluteus maximus, with a chemical dye that glows yellow when exposed to light from an ultraviolet lamp. This helps locate the exact area of the buttock that gets its blood supply from the injected artery. The area is carefully removed along with the artery and vein supplying it, and the gap in the buttock is closed, leaving only a small hollow. The graft is then sewn in place on the chest to make a new breast, and its artery and vein are plugged into chest blood vessels using a microscope to make the connections.

There are many potential problems. The flap tissue can die from a failure in the blood supply. Sometimes, the flap does not form into a breast shape. Even when it does, once the swelling goes down, the graft can turn out to be too large or too small or in the wrong position, all of which are difficult or impossible to adjust. The only really good thing that can be said of this operation is that, if it fails for any reason, the transplanted tissue can be removed from its place on the chest and thrown away, and there's no real harm done. Of course, you would have a hollow appearance in your behind.

But if you're bound and determined (and crazy), a hunk can be taken from the other side and the procedure tried again. At least you would have a balanced behind.

The real downside is that some doctors who perform this procedure are not very good at it. Even when done by the best, the operation can typically take 12 hours, which significantly increases the risk of dangerous clots and other complications from being under anesthesia for so long. Overall, there is a 10 percent chance that the transplanted tissue will die in the days and weeks after surgery. Another operation is then necessary to remove the black, dead mass. There are few more discouraging sounds a patient can hear than her surgeon switching from his "trust-me, it will be great" routine before the operation to his glum "these things happen, I'm sorry" story afterward.

Short-Rectus Flaps

In the short-rectus flap operation, a short upper segment of one or both rectus muscles—the pair of muscles that run down the midline of the abdomen—is transferred to the chest through a tunnel under the skin. The flap of muscle, sometimes along with some skin and fat, is then shaped into a breast and sewn in place. If needed, a saline-filled implant can be inserted underneath. Though not as fraught with danger as the TRAM flap operation, this procedure has its downside as well. It is touted as a substitute for the back muscle transfer when that is not available, but it is greatly inferior. The rectus muscle is thicker and far narrower than the back muscle, so it covers a much smaller area of the chest, and the results tend to look bulkier than those of the back muscle procedure. In addition, it has the same problems with tissue death, size, shape, position, and scarring as the other tissue transfers. Finally, because most women will not be able to do sit-ups after the abdominal surgery, the biggest worry about this operation is the potential for chronic back pain.

As in other procedures, the operation begins with the surgeon outlining the part of the muscle and skin to be transferred. The pocket that will receive the flap, as well as the bottom fold of the breast to be rebuilt, is mapped out. The initial incision is made to free the flap of abdominal skin, fat, and muscle, leaving it attached only to the upper part of the rectus muscle. Next, the skin is raised from the mastectomized side, and a pocket is made to accept the transferred tissue. A tunnel under the skin is created connecting the chest to the flap of tissue to be transferred. Finally, the flap is passed through the tunnel into the chest and sewn in place. If enough skin and fat have been brought with the muscle, they can be shaped into a breast. Otherwise, a small saline implant is put under the muscle temporarily. (After the chest has healed three months later, a full-size implant can be substituted.) Patients usually go home on the second day after surgery and can resume light activities. Sutures are removed after a week, and strenuous activities must be avoided for three weeks.

The TRAM Flap

And now we come again to the infamous TRAM flap: the triumph of the plastic surgeon's mania for proving it's possible to move anything anywhere even if it flies in the face of common sense. I am spending so much time talking about this operation simply because it makes me quite angry even to hear that it is being done.

The TRAM flap requires the full or near-full length of rectus muscle that extends from the chest to the pubic bone and a far larger flap of attached skin and fat, from the belly. (For that reason it is sometimes called the long-rectus flap procedure.) Many doctors try to sell the operation to patients by telling them that a side benefit of the technique is a tummy tuck, though in fact because of bulging at the ends of the hip-to-hip scar that is left—what some plastic surgeons refer to as "dog ears"—the waist paradoxically grows in size. What's more, the operation usually produces an ugly, scarred, misshapen blob of wide-pored, hairy, abdominal flab that sits bunched up on the chest like it had just come out of a crenellated Jell-O® mold. Afterward, many women bitterly regret that they opted for this procedure instead of a simple implant or even instead of doing nothing.

There's more. People have died from blood vessel obstructions and blockages to the lungs caused by fiddling around with all that abdominal fat. In up to ten percent of patients, part of the TRAM flap turns black and dies within the first few days as a result of poor circulation and must be removed. For one in ten patients, problems don't surface for three months. Then it becomes apparent that the amount of flesh and fat transplanted isn't quite right, and the patient must go through another operation to reduce or enlarge the breast size. And that becomes more risky because then the blood supply is being tinkered with, which is very tenuous in TRAM flaps. And even if the whole flap does not die, the part that was fat may melt away. And if it does, the result will be a breast that's too small. I have read reports in medical journals by people who've performed a TRAM flap where the breast ended up too small, and they just blithely state, "So we went back a couple of months later and put in a small implant."

The technique leaves behind no supporting gristle layer or muscle in the lower abdomen. Because most patients won't be able to do sit-ups and other abdominal exercises, they cannot protect against or relieve back pain. Patients are also left utterly vulnerable to hernia, in which the intestine pushes through the peritoneum, the abdominal lining. The incidence of hernia after this operation is high: eight to ten percent over a few years. And those hernias are horrible. The general surgeons hate them because they are nearly impossible to fix, as there's no longer any supportive muscle or gristle.

To protect against hernias, some doctors, when doing the TRAM flap, are now putting in a plastic mesh to help keep the patient's innards in. The only problem is that meshes get old. After a few years they tend to get brittle and fragment. So if a woman with a mesh does get a hernia years later and doctors go in to repair it, they often find artificial mesh all over the place that is bound to the muscle, the scar tissue, and even to the peritoneum and intestines. And if it gets infected, real problems result. Infections are hard to get rid of because they mix in with the plastic mesh. The peritoneum would have to be taken out and the bowel exposed or removed. The truly ironic part about all this is that even if these problems don't happen, we still have patients walking around with artificial meshes in their bodies when the whole come-on for the procedure was to avoid artificial implantation.

Which leads me to ask, Why would anyone take a chance on any of those things happening in order to create a new breast? From an objective point of view, the benefits do not outweigh the risks. It has been suggested that the reason TRAM flaps are done so often is that many plastic surgeons are not very busy and they get paid three times more to do TRAMs than simple implantations. I hope that is not true but insurance company payments may be more of a driving force on what is done in medicine than anybody quite realizes.

Nipple Reconstruction

Of course, when a woman has her breast removed, the nipple goes, too. So women having breast reconstruction usually, but not always, wish to have a nipple reconstructed as well. Sometimes during mastectomy, a woman's own nipple and areola can be preserved by grafting it on to the patient's abdomen or thigh for at least six months. Unfortunately, such transfers often are too traumatic on the tissue, and the nipple undergoes a change in shape and color that renders it shrunken and unusable. Nipples stored temporarily in a skin bank at low temperatures hold up better and can produce excellent results. Unfortunately, there are so few skin banks that this is often impractical.

Among the many imaginative ways to reconstruct the nipple and surrounding areola include grafts from tissue surrounding the vagina; from the thigh, ear, or toe tip; or even from part of the healthy nipple. Unfortunately, halving the normal nipple and transferring it to the reconstructed side sometimes results in shriveled, scarred nipples on both sides.

Grafts from the ear are too pale; vaginal skin tends to become too dark. Toe grafts too often still resemble toes, as toeprints remain. I've found that the best way to rebuild a nipple is to fashion one from a small block of tissue from the labium majus, the fleshy outer border of the vaginal opening. For the areola, skin from the inner thigh or a graft from the healthy breast usually works very well.

Women worry that their graft sites will be painful, but in truth there's hardly any discomfort during or after surgery. The stitches used in the perineum and groin are the melting kind and do not have to be removed. Sensory nerves grow easily into the grafts, but those responsible for erotic signals do not seem to regenerate. That means that the new nipple will have near-normal skin sensation but will not convey sexual sensations. Even when grafts are not possible, as a last resort a nipple and areola can be tattooed on the breast. Remember, although reconstructed breasts should look and feel as natural as possible in the nude, the bottom-line goal is to fashion breasts that appear natural when a bra is worn. This at least enables women to wear low-cut dresses and bathing suits.

As in most other aspects of breast reconstruction and augmentation, the simplest solutions are often the best. Every day, women are talked into getting complicated flaps as a way of avoiding implants. In time, many (if not most) wish that they had opted for a saline-filled implant, which, as Chapter 5 makes clear, is the simplest solution. Don't forget that with saline, even if the implant should turn completely to mud, it can be removed in five minutes with a drop of novocaine, and the woman is no worse off medically than she was when it was put in.

4

The Silicone Gel Mess

Now the Public Knows What Doctors Knew All Along

I first realized that all silicone gel–filled implants leak when I returned from a six-week trip in 1972 and discovered that I had inadvertently left one on my leather-top desk at the office while I was away. To my surprise, there was a greasy circle under the implant.

In those days I was a full-time assistant professor of surgery at New York Hospital/Cornell Medical Center. As an employee, I never purchased implants; the hospital did. But I did know the sales representative from Dow Corning, who regularly came by to take orders. The next time I ran into him, I asked about the greasy circle the gel implant had left on my desk. He seemed rather taken aback and offered no explanation. He did, however, agree to a little experiment. We took a new silicone gel–filled implant and put it on a metal-top desk. Then we covered it with a small empty box, which we taped down so it would not be disturbed. At the end of two weeks, when the Dow representative returned, we lifted up the box. There was without a question a greasy spot on the desk; even the surface of the implant felt greasy. I asked him to check back with the people at Dow. He later reported back to me that they were unaware of this problem, and I gathered that they were uninterested, though I wasn't certain that he had actually talked to anyone senior. When I pressed the matter, Dow always came up with some specious answer, such as that maybe I had cleaned the implant and forgotten to wash the soap off. Nobody at Dow seemed to care, and its sales continued to increase every month.

Silicone "Bleed"

Today, it's clear that Dow was aware that its implants bled silicone gel. That came out in 1992 in the midst of FDA deliberations on the safety of silicone gel–filled breast implants. The FDA hearings had led to the public release in February 1992 of thousands of pages of Dow's internal documents. Many of the memos focused on implants developed in the 1970s that were made with a thinner gel and a thinner outer envelope so they would feel more natural. However, the memos suggest that there was a concern as to whether the thinner gel also may have made the silicone more prone to breaking down to a liquid, which tended to "bleed" or "sweat" through the thinner silicone casing. As pointed out by a congressional staff report of the human resources and intergovernmental relations subcommittee released in January 1993, the memos suggested that Dow worried more about the gel bleed problem hurting sales than about the possibility that it might be harmful to patients. In fact, Dow was so concerned about silicone bleeding during sales displays that one Dow memo advised salesmen to wash the implants before showing them to doctors lest their greasy feel turn doctors off. It stated that washing was necessary because bleeding tended to occur the day after the implants were handled. There was no show of concern that it would follow that the implant would also bleed silicone inside the patient.

In fact, the finding that silicone gel–filled implants still bled silicone was one of the FDA's prime concerns when it first asked for a voluntary moratorium on their use in January 1992. The agency stated then that the significance of silicone bleed would become clear only after further studies. But clinical observations certainly suggest that gel bleed leads to the formation of scar tissue that actually weaves its way around each molecule of liquid silicone that escapes from the implant. The result is not just a hardened capsule of scar tissue around the implant itself but also tough capsules around each silicone particle. These can form lumps, which sometimes contain microscopic calcium deposits, that are virtually indistinguishable from cancerous tumors except after they're surgically removed at biopsy and analyzed.

Dow was not the only implant maker that realized very early that its products bled silicone. The government's investigation of silicone gel–filled implants also revealed a memo showing that, as early as April 1977, Medical Engineering Corporation's scientific affairs committee intimated that silicone bleeding into the surrounding body tissue could someday lead the FDA to remove silicone gel implants from the market.

Dow's Internal Memos

Information disclosed by implant makers has been revealing, provocative, and even shocking. The February, 1992, public release of internal documents by Dow Corning, for instance, showed that as far back as the mid-1970s, it was marketing implants before animal safety studies were completed and even while some were linking implants with risks of immune disorders. Other preliminary animal studies at the time had suggested that the silicone could migrate or cause other problems. In 1985, an internal Dow memo warned that the results of long-term safety testing of their implants' silicone shells had been adequate but that testing of the gel was not. In fact, most of Dow's safety claims, a Dow document states, had been based solely on a two-year study of dogs.

Documents show that Dow's scientists were concerned that company spokesmen were misleading doctors about the safety of its implants. For example, Chuck Leach, a marketing executive, wrote in a 1977 memorandum that at a conference of plastic surgeons he spoke "with crossed fingers" of studies on gel migration and capsular contracture. He now says that he meant he was hopeful that Dow would build upon preliminary studies that were under way. However, he was not as optimistic in the 1977 memo: "As best I can tell, we have not taken significant action ... except for a halfhearted low priority program."

Blasé FDA

In fact, the FDA itself showed only a halfhearted interest in whether silicone gel–filled implants were safe. True, the FDA proposed in 1982 that manufacturers submit safety and efficacy studies. But the agency let nine years go by—and let perhaps a million more women get the implants—before officially calling for safety data. Even more shocking is that in 1991, when newly appointed FDA chief Dr. David Kessler told his underlings that he did not intend to let another anniversary of inactivity go by, FDA scientists confided in him that they had their doubts that adequate safety studies had ever been done. There was concern among some scientific advisors that, if safety data were lacking, Kessler would have no choice but to ban silicone gel–filled implants—a concern that reflects a head-in-the-sand attitude among top people at the FDA. But to Kessler's credit, he dismissed the notion that he leave gel-filled implants alone. Kessler recalls: "My feeling was that 10 years was long enough and that it was time to call for the data."

Of course, many implant makers and plastic surgeons were, in fact, busy conducting studies of their own in a race to develop new designs that they could market as more pleasing or less prone to hardening than the latest model of competitors. But according to the congressional report, in 1989 one plastic surgeon in private practice wrote to the FDA to blow the whistle on what he said had become "the custom and practice" among plastic surgeons and implant makers of using women as guinea pigs in unsanctioned studies. He charged that manufacturers routinely modify their implants on the basis of ideas of surgeons and then provide these custom-made prototypes to doctors who would try them out on patients to see how well they worked, even when no animal studies were done first. He wrote that he had stopped the practice because he felt that it was unethical. Besides, he told the FDA, his 20 to 25 percent complication rate was unjustifiably high, according to the congressional report.

Doctors Didn't Care

Studies that should have sounded an alarm about silicone implants were drowned out by the enthusiastic reports published in the medical journals and discussed at conferences. The surgical community filled volumes of pages and endless meetings with praise for implants. Aside from problems such as painful hardening, serious complications were only rarely reported on at length. Those who wrote in the journals, wrote books, or spoke out in professional meetings about the dangers of bleeding implants and liquid silicone were ignored and, if they persisted, were shunned. I have had personal experience, and it is neither pleasant nor easy. Even so, everyone knew by the mid-1970s that silicone bleed was a reality, but no one wanted to deal with it. Most plastic surgeons who took the time even to consider switching to saline implants apparently dismissed the idea because it was too much trouble to learn how to use them, and, after all, no one had proved that liquid silicone did any harm. In fact, at conferences the notion of silicone traveling in the body was made light of. During one meeting in Washington, D.C., as late as 1992, a chief of plastic surgery commented that toothpaste contains silicone; he asked if I wanted people to stop brushing their teeth.

This is typical of the deliberate misinformation put out by the proponents of silicone gel–filled implants. They do not mention that the amount of silicone in toothpaste is absolutely insignificant compared to that released from implants. They ignore the fact that any silicone in toothpaste enters only the digestive tract and is eventually eliminated, whereas the silicone sweating out of silicone gel–filled implants enters the bloodstream and lymph system, through which it surely invades the body's organs. You can see how difficult it is to argue with these people even to this day. I suppose it is unreasonable to expect that those who in the past were unwilling to admit that they were wrong in front of their colleagues would now be willing to do so in front of two million women waiting to sue.

Unpublished Studies

The charade has been kept alive by manufacturers who released results of studies that yielded only favorable results. Dow Corning data on silicone gel–breakdown and other problems were withheld from the FDA and from publication in medical journals, according to federal investigators. Medical Engineering Corporation, the company that was sold to Bristol-Myers Squibb, did not always disclose the results of research that was potentially damaging either. In fact, documents gathered by congressional investigators suggest Medical Engineering tried to cover them up. After a 1978 memo discussing studies of dogs implicated silicone gel–filled implants in bleeding, pneumonia, and lesions of the large intestines, the response of Medical Engineering was, "Sacrifice dogs ASAP." A year later, Medical Engineering responded to a letter about animal maintenance costs with a note recommending, "Kill dogs; forget organs."

Despite the coverups and unpublished articles, by 1982 the FDA had heard enough unanswered questions about silicone implants that it took action. It published, in the government periodical *The Federal Register*, a proposed rule requiring manufacturers to undertake safety and efficacy studies. As it turns out, the potential risks the FDA pointed to were virtually the same that ten years later led the agency to pull gel-filled implants from the market. Yet plastic surgeons continued unabatedly to assure their patients that the gel implants they were placing behind their breasts were safe. Here's a quick summary of what was known and when.

Hardening Breast Implants

Since the 1960s, hundreds of reports have shown that scar tissue forms around implants, causing pain as it hardens and contracting in as many as 74 percent of women with gel implants. Slight hardening may barely be noticed; in the worst cases, implants became as hard as rocks. For many years, doctors have tried to crack the capsule shells by squeezing them manually, a procedure doctors call "closed capsulotomy" in front of patients and "popping" among themselves. It's quite a painful procedure because, by lacing one's fingers together and compressing the implant with both palms, a big, orthopedic-type plastic surgeon can develop an enormous amount of pressure. Most plastic surgeons have abandoned this technique for many reasons, including, by poetic justice, back injuries and sprained thumbs they sustained while performing this worthless procedure.

Studies suggest that complications, such as bleeding and blood clot formation, arise in 12 to 16 percent of closed capsulotomies. What's more, the capsules get hard again 67 percent of the time as the crack in the capsule closes up, sometimes as soon as ten days. Even if the capsule does stay open, part of the implant would sometimes bulge out, producing a kind of dumbbell effect. But the worst thing that could happen would be that the silicone implant would burst, releasing large amounts of silicone into the surrounding body tissue, some of which would wander throughout the body.

It's a serious event when a silicone gel–filled implant bursts; doctors must operate and either remove wide areas of breast tissue contaminated by silicone or try suctioning it out, which is not very effective. Most patients with silicone in soft tissue are left with some residual silicone that can leave breasts chronically tender and inflamed.

In "open capsulotomy," the breasts are reoperated on, the capsules are broken up using a scalpel, and the implants are replaced. Even this procedure is not a good idea if gel-filled implants have been used. Breaking up those capsules, which invariably contain a large amount of sweated silicone, releases silicone into the body. Such implants and their capsules must be removed intact. Even after surgery, severe tightness returns for somewhere between 25 and 89 percent of patients if a gel-filled implant is used. It goes without saying that if an implant is put back, it should be one that's filled with saline.

Surgeons have tried nearly everything to prevent the hardening process, from different implant shapes and textures to balms, antibiotics, and steroids, but the problem has persisted. Only saline implants have worked predictably (see Chapter 5). By 1990, plastic surgeons were so forlorn that some even suggested that breast hardening was something to strive for. "We're all aware of patients who have contracture . . . on only one side . . . but complain about the still soft breast," wrote one leading plastic surgeon in a 1990 medical journal article. "Many women prefer the firmer breast because of better projection."

Leakage

In 1978, researchers at an FDA advisory panel meeting on breast implants discussed research results suggesting that silicone might seep out of even intact gel implants. It was a topic of considerable interest, federal investigators recall, considering that, at the time, patients were being told that only a full-blown rupture—caused, say, by a car accident— could release silicone from their implants. The fact is that manufacturers never really got very excited about whether a gel-filled implant formed a hole and released the gel because they felt the gel wasn't going anywhere. Ten years later, however, FDA scientists were back at the panel room sifting through studies suggesting that silicone that seeps out of implants can migrate throughout the body and cause breast deformities, skin ulceration, burning sensation and pain, enlarged lymph nodes, palpable masses, respiratory distress, and immune disorders.

Problems with implants developing holes have since been traced to the implant's type of shell, whether clear or opaque. The clear-shell implants look better when the implant is sitting on the table. They have kind of a beauty to them. They're crystal clear, and the light refracts through them a little bit like a diamond. However, under a microscope you can see that their surfaces are rough. What's more, where rough, wrinkled surfaces rub against each other, there's a propensity to wear away a hole. The opaque shells, on the other hand, have a surface that is rather drab to the naked eye but looks very smooth under a microscope and so tends not to form holes, making it far superior. Surgeons who read their monthly copy of *Plastic and Reconstructive Surgery* should know this fact. Still, manufacturers have kept marketing the clear-shelled implants, probably because they're so much prettier and plastic surgeons have continued to use them.

Autoimmune Disease

In February 1975, an internal Dow Corning document first raised concerns about inflammatory reactions to implants in animal studies. It was unclear whether the reaction was a result of the implant or the technique used, but apparently the findings did not stop Dow from continuing to market the implants. It was not until 1979 that the first published studies appeared linking gel implants to immune diseases. In 1982, investigators reported an association with rheumatoid arthritis and lupus, the latter being a disorder in which the body's immune system attacks the body's own tissues. The following year a researcher reported on a patient who developed joint pain, swollen lymph nodes, weight loss, and weakness after one of her gel implants ruptured; she recovered after implant removal.

By March 1990 there were 90 cases reported of various types of autoimmune diseases in patients with silicone gel–filled implants, including some with crippling connective tissue diseases such as scleroderma, which causes thickening of the skin and internal organs. However, in December 1992 a task force from the plastic surgical and rheumatological communities published a consensus statement finding that there is insufficient information "to implicate silicone implants in scleroderma-like disorders or any other autoimmune disease." Only large-scale scientific studies will answer the question, but the final study results may not be in until 1997.

Cancer

A two-year study in rats of two kinds of silicone gel implants by Dow Corning in 1988 was offered to the FDA as evidence that implants were safe. In fact, some of the rats developed fibrosarcomas, a type of tumor that Dow dismissed as irrelevant, saying that it does not occur in humans. However, one FDA reviewer expressed concern about the malignant tumors found in approximately one-fourth of the rats. Many of those tumors had spread to the lungs, liver, and other organs. What's more, the FDA reviewer quoted scientists who reported that such tumors had been detected in humans.

In an internal memo written in March 1990, an FDA pharmacologist expressed concern that silicone breast implants that were covered with polyurethane foam might pose a cancer risk. Many thousands of women had been implanted with those types of implants, one of the most popular models being the Même, which was sold by Surgitek, a subsidiary of Bristol-Myers Squibb (as you may recall from Chapter 1). On the basis of two studies conducted for Surgitek on the breakdown of foam into a substance called TDA, a known animal carcinogen, the FDA pharmacologist estimated that the lifetime cancer risk could run as high as 180 in 1 million. Still, it was not until mid-April 1991, when the FDA was issuing its directive giving makers of all breast implants 90 days to provide safety studies, that the FDA's concerns about foam-covered implants and TDA were made public. What's more, it was the *New York Times*, not the FDA, that reported the startling revelation. Four days later, Bristol-Myers Squibb announced it was voluntarily suspending shipments of its polyurethane foam–covered implants until the FDA had an opportunity to review all the relevant data.

As it turned out, the concern was bolstered by more than studies of rats. On June 4, 1991, Aegis Analytical Laboratories in Nashville gave the FDA the results of a study it had done at Surgitek's request finding TDA in the breast milk of a woman with polyurethane-covered implants. Surgitek officials had argued that the finding was inaccurate, though a third-party expert in forensic toxicology retained by Surgitek to review the results had confirmed that the laboratory methods were "accurate and appropriate," according to Aegis.

As for other types of gel implants, two studies published in 1992 suggest that after ten years, at least, there is no increase in breast cancer risk from implants. But even if silicone gel implants don't cause cancer, might they not increase a woman's cancer risk by undermining cancer detection tests? As far back as 1977, scientists first voiced their concern that gel-filled implants obscured mammography, or breast X rays, making it more difficult to detect tiny tumors. In 1978, investigators reported in *Plastic and Reconstructive Surgery* that gel implants made it possible to visualize only about 25 percent of the breast. Many physicians and even radiologists assumed that implants rendered mammographic studies practically useless. It wasn't until September 1988 that investigators at the Oregon Health Sciences University in Portland came up with a solution. Their positioning technique enabled specially trained mammographers to pull the breast tissue over and in front of the implant long enough to take the X rays. Still, if a woman's breasts are firm or hard because of contracture, it is difficult to compress the breast adequately. (See Chapter 6 for a full discussion of imaging techniques for women with implants.)

The Hidden Scandal

With all these studies on the risks of silicone gel–filled implants, it's a mystery that doctors didn't just throw these implants in the garbage. But what's more scandalous is that the public didn't know there were problems until now. Americans have been misled about gel-filled implants for at least 15 years. All you have to do is read the public information brochure *Straight Talk ... About Breast Implants*, which is published by the American Society of Plastic and Reconstructive Surgeons (ASPRS), the official professional organization of plastic surgeons, and endorsed by the American Society for Aesthetic Plastic Surgery, an offshoot organization. Primarily used in 1990 and 1991, when gel implants were being put in some 13,000 women a month, the 13-page pamphlet purports to contain the "state of medical knowledge." It even gives the impression that it serves as a kind of informed-consent form as it includes a page for patients to sign, stating that they've read the pamphlet and that their doctors have answered all their questions satisfactorily. A close read of the pamphlet, however, shows that it contains information that we know today is clearly false. For instance, the brochure claims that capsular contracture affects "one out of ten women," whereas even the medical literature at the time reported 30 to 40 percent contracture rates, a figure that is actually much too low for gel-filled implants.

The brochure also states that "loose silicone does not appear to be a health risk" and suggests that the longevity of breast implants can be compared to "the kidney, heart, eyes or any other body part." In describing "fuzzy" or polyurethane covered implants, the brochure states that, although no health risks from the breakdown of the foam have been identified, it is not known what effect it may have over a lifetime. In fact, by 1989, investigators had reported studies in which the foam broke down to TDA, a chemical listed as a cause of cancer in animals and a possible carcinogen for humans. And at least six studies published between 1982 and 1988 reported a variety of complications, such as infection, unusual allergic reaction, and severe breast pain.

Medical Misinformation

There are other examples of misinformation perpetu-
ated in part by the ASPRS. The society first went on the
offensive in October 1991, not long after congressional hearings aired potential problems with silicone gel implants.
Breast implantation was at that time, after all, one of the
most common procedures in plastic surgery in the United
States. Though it funded some research on silicone gel–filled
implants, the ASPRS seemed chiefly interested in financing
an extensive lobbying campaign aimed at putting pressure
on the government to curb its regulatory actions. It did this
by charging an additional assessment of $1,050 over a three-
year period beginning in the fall of 1991 to each of its
members. These assessments were mandatory to maintain
membership.

The ASPRS had said some of the donations would go to
fund new research into breast implants and some, through its
political action committee PlastyPac, would go to legislators
"who have demonstrated a sympathetic interest" in the availability of breast implants and to express the society's "support and gratitude." As noted in Chapter 1, by the first quarter
of 1993 about $1 million had been spent on national lobbying
and "individual members' government efforts."

The ASPRS paid for or "encouraged" women to fly to
Washington to lobby their senators and congressmen about
the importance of breast implants. It also orchestrated a
letter-writing campaign by more than 20,000 plastic surgeons,
nurses and patients to Congress and the FDA. According to
the recently released congressional staff report, as a result of
such lobbying, more than 200 congressmen and senators

wrote to FDA commissioner Kessler advising him to keep implants on the market.

Targeting Kessler

When Kessler defied them by calling for a voluntary moratorium on breast implants in January 1992, key ASPRS members sought reasons why he and several members of the FDA advisory panel should abstain from the decision-making process. The society had hired three lobbying firms, assembling a team that included three lobbyists with ties to the Bush administration and three with ties to the FDA. They reportedly arranged various telephone conversations between the ASPRS and Louis Sullivan, Secretary of the U.S. Department of Health and Human Services, and with staff members of Vice President Dan Quayle's Competitiveness Council. But in the end, only Dr. Norman Anderson, former chair of the FDA advisory committee, was stripped of his vote, ostensibly because he had told the press of his concerns about silicone gel–filled implants, which, the FDA maintained, brought his objectivity into question.

FDA Downplays Risks

Even after Kessler announced in April 1992 that silicone gel–filled breast implants would be available only under tightly controlled clinical studies, the ASPRS kept up its lobbying efforts, this time to influence the FDA to downplay the risks of the implants. The ASPRS's target was the FDA's new,

The Truth about Breast Implants

mandatory informed-consent form, a five-page document that, Kessler ruled, doctors had to walk patients through as a way of outlining the risks involved in gel implants and the implantation procedure. To the ASPRS, the informed-consent document was unnecessarily alarming and exposed physicians to possible litigation. On June 5, 1992, the executive director of the ASPRS wrote to Dr. Alan Anderson, the acting director of the FDA's office of device evaluation, objecting to key points in the FDA's informed-consent form and to suggest changes. His letter was followed two weeks later by one from Dr. James Todd, the executive vice president of the American Medical Association, in support of some of ASPRS's complaints. The society's efforts culminated in a telephone conference call in mid-July with the ASPRS and three top FDA officials. Among other requests, the ASPRS asked that the FDA do the following:

- Delete the FDA's statement that "although there is no evidence that silicone used in breast implants causes cancer in humans, the possibility has not been ruled out" and replace it with "There is no evidence that silicone used in breast implants causes cancer in humans." (The FDA's final version follows the ASPRS's lead but retains in a follow-up sentence that the possibility of cancer cannot be ruled out.)

- Delete the warning that implantation "may interfere with a woman's ability to nurse her baby ..." and replace it with "There is no evidence that breast implants interfere with lactation and many women with implants have successfully nursed." (The FDA's final version begins, "Many women with breast implants have nursed their babies successfully," and only later states that implant surgery "could theoretically" interfere with breastfeeding.)

- Delete language that there was insufficient evidence to determine the relationship of implants to birth defects and replace it with a statement that there is no evidence that breast implants can lead to birth defects. (The FDA's final version begins, "Preliminary animal studies show no evidence that birth defects are caused by breast implants," and is followed up by a statement that further studies are needed to rule out the possibility for humans.)

- Delete the statement that doctors "must not" perform closed capsulotomy, the brute-force method for cracking capsules by pressing forcefully on the chest, and replace it with: "While the FDA and manufacturers recommend against closed capsulotomy ... some physicians based on clinical experience feel that closed capsulotomy is an appropriate treatment in some patients. However, patients must understand that closed capsulotomy could cause an implant to break and that would require surgery to replace the implants." (The FDA's final version closely follows the ASPRS's and goes even further by dropping the statement that the FDA recommends against the procedure.)

- Delete any statement suggesting that there was not adequate scientific evidence of the safety and effectiveness of silicone gel–filled implants. (The FDA stuck to its guns in the final version, stating, "The [FDA] is concerned that there is not enough information about possible health problems from the use of these devices.")

- Delete statements to the effect that no one really knows how many women have had problems with their silicone gel–filled breast implants. (The FDA's final version: "Although there are risks and complications of having breast implants, most women implanted have had satisfactory results.")

Bureaucratic Lunacy

In a special bulletin to its membership, the ASPRS calls the changes "one of ASPRS' greatest victories in the breast implant controversy to date." The newsletter continues, "The alarmist language of the original document has been significantly diminished and replaced with a more realistic document that spells out what is actually known about breast implants, instead of speculation about possible risks." For its part, the FDA says the changes were made as a necessary compromise, noting that a two-year joint effort with plastic surgeons, consumer's groups, and implant manufacturers failed completely to come up with simple pamphlets that were to be distributed voluntarily. The society also came up with its own addendum to the FDA's informed-consent document that states, "It is the position of [ASPRS] that the FDA-mandated document overstates the risks" of gel-filled implants. It then lists diluted warnings—for major disorders such as cancer, rheumatic disorders, and birth defects—under the heading "Speculative long-term risks."

The Silicone Gel Mess

It is probably more a matter of bureaucratic lunacy than of lobbying efforts that more than a year after the FDA's restrictions on silicone gel implants, virtually any woman who wants a silicone gel implant for breast enlargement can still get one with ease. The recent congressional subcommittee staff report shows that the FDA has had virtually no role in monitoring the use of gel implants. Physicians must merely sign a form stating that silicone breast implants are necessary because saline implants are "unsuitable." Moreover, according to the report, doctors are not required to document whether implants are necessary for reconstruction or to correct a deformity. Any doctor, then, who believes that silicone implants are better than saline implants is able to continue to use gel implants, the report concludes, and any doctor who believes small breasts are "a deformity" can continue to do breast enlargement surgery with gel implants.

Manufacturers of silicone gel implants and the doctors who use them take the position that as long as there is no way to prove that silicone gel implants cause birth defects, problems with breastfeeding, or immune disorders, any suggestion that they do is just government interference. But, in my view, it should not be left to the government to prove that something is harmful; rather, doctors should prove that materials they use are safe. And, because there isn't much that anyone can say for sure about silicone gel–filled implants, they simply should not be used. In today's climate, surgeons who use gel-filled implants have surely taken leave of their senses and, when they have problems, should not be surprised when they are sued.

The argument becomes even more egregious in the knowledge that implants filled with harmless saltwater are available. What will manufacturers of silicone gel implants say if 20 years from now it's absolutely proved that silicone implants caused damage? They'll say how sorry they were and that they didn't know better, and they're going to be exactly like the cigarette companies. There won't be a dime's worth of difference. Furthermore, plastic surgeons will tell every new patient that they never used gel-filled implants, and indeed, that they are long-time experts in the use of saline-filled implants. It will be harder to find an ex-gel·user than an ex-communist in Russia. We are actually seeing this phenomenon already.

Having Silicone Gel–Filled Implants Removed

I believe that silicone in liquid form may act as a catalyst for harmful reactions to take place inside the body. Natural and synthetic substances that don't ordinarily combine might find a way to link up in the presence of liquid silicone. Silicone may, for instance, act as a surface on which these other chemical reactions take place to cause immune disorders, inflammation, and other health problems. We know that silicone gel–filled implants bleed liquid silicone molecule by molecule. That means that the surface area of silicone inside the body continues to grow over time as more silicone molecules escape from the implant into the tissues. With every day that goes by, more silicone escapes, and the greater the risk that something will go wrong. If that's so, then removing the implant—the source of the liquid silicone—should alleviate any present disease or reduce the chance of developing problems.

And indeed, well-done scientific studies are beginning to support that notion. In October 1992, Dr. William Shaw, a plastic surgeon at the University of California at Los Angeles, reported at a symposium sponsored by the American Medical Association in Marina Del Ray, California, that patients with silicone gel–filled breast implants who had local and systemic medical problems improved after their implants were removed. Among 150 patients, 90 percent of the local complaints, such as discomfort in the chest, were relieved or substantially improved, and 70 percent of systemic symptoms such as chronic fatigue or joint pain, improved. It's not clear precisely why the women improved, says Shaw, but he suspects that one reason may be that their silicone gel–filled implants were causing some kind of chronic inflammatory reaction.

Symptoms Disappear

At a subcommittee hearing in December 1990, Dr. Frank Vasey, a professor of medicine at the University of South Florida, testified that he had recommended that 18 patients who had complained of major problems such as lupus, scleroderma, arthritis, and severe muscle pain consider having their gel-filled implants removed. Three months to two years later, all but two of the women had significantly improved, and two of the most seriously ill patients appeared to be cured. By March 1992, Vasey had data on 50 breast implant patients with connective tissue and immune system

The Truth about Breast Implants

complaints, 33 of whom chose to have their implants removed. His findings: in 25 (76 percent) of these women, symptoms improved or disappeared in an average of 22 months. Now Vasey has data on 500 women that back up his initial observations that symptoms subside after gel-filled implants are removed. Vasey says critics may argue that at least some of these women may be simply experiencing "spontaneous remission" of their symptoms for reasons unrelated to their implant removal, but so far no studies have contradicted his clinical observations. This could be powerful supporting evidence that the silicone is causing these diseases. And in lawsuits, it may even be considered to be *res ipse loquitur*: "the thing speaks for itself."

In fact, in medical journals doctors are beginning to be told that they may be liable if they do not counsel women about removing their silicone gel–filled implants. In a July 1992 article in the state medical journal *Minnesota Medicine*, Keith Halleland, a Minneapolis lawyer, wrote in a column titled "Medicine Law and Policy" that physicians may be open to litigation if a patient who experiences apparently implant-related health problems can show that she would have had the implants removed had she received complete advice regarding the risks of keeping them in place. Halleland suggests three potential defenses doctors may use to counter patients' claims of negligence for failing to remove silicone gel–filled implants. First, he says, physicians may maintain that they warned their patients and that they chose to ignore the advice. Second, Halleland writes, the physician may rely on available FDA and manufacturer recommendations that support the physician's advice. Finally, there's always the statute of limitations, Halleland notes, that in Minnesota may bar a claim if more than two years have elapsed since the date of treatment. Other states have similar statutes.

Change Them All

When the FDA restricted the use of gel–filled implants, it advised women who are not having any medical problems with their implants not to have them removed. But in medicine, we always have to consider the quality of life. It's not of any physiological value to live forever if it means living in fear and misery. So, if a woman is constantly wondering what these things are doing to her and is constantly aware that these implants are in her chest, then it seems to me that it doesn't make sense to keep them. According to a report by the government watchdog agency the Government Accounting Office, most government and private insurers will pay for the removal of silicone breast implants, even those done for solely cosmetic reasons. But insurers do require that the patient's physician determine that the procedure is medically necessary. Similarly, Dow Corning will reimburse part of the cost for implant removal under certain conditions. And women may wish to contact Bristol-Myers Squibb to ask under what circumstances it or its subsidiary companies that dealt in implants will help pay for removal of breast implants. Women may have to be persistent, however, in seeking answers to their questions.

Because saline implants are an alternative, and because changing implants is simple and can often be done under local anaesthesia, it makes common sense to change them all. Of course, doctors have to remove any leaked silicone and

scar capsule before putting in a saline-filled implant. However, the risks involved in the operation of substituting saline
for silicone gel implants—though they are rare and not life
threatening—have to be weighed. As you will see in Chapter
5, I feel that those risks are well worth taking.

5

The Saline Solution

The Simplest Choice
Is Best

Now that the public knows what plastic surgeons and makers of silicone gel–filled implants have kept under wraps for so long, the question I hear most from patients is, "If saline-filled implants are so safe, why wasn't everyone using them all along?"

Most plastic surgeons don't want you to hear the answer. Saline-filled implants have been available for nearly 20 years. Yet doctors have used them in only 10 to 15 percent of breast reconstruction and augmentation procedures. For virtually all the rest they chose silicone gel–filled implants, even though they knew full-well that gel-filled implants leach wayward silicone, leaving a trail of unanswered questions about the consequences. If asked why they didn't switch to saline-filled implants, most plastic surgeons will put on their most earnest faces, lace their fingers, look you in the eyes, and recite tired, misleading excuses such as, "Saline-filled implants leak." They won't tell you that design improvements more than 15 years ago largely solved leakage problems.

The Truth about Saline-Filled Implants

Back in the mid-1970s, saline-filled implants that were largely handmade often had shells that were too thin in places or had defective valves, which led to leaks in as many as three out of four implants after a few months. Today only 1 in 300 or 400 leak, as opposed to gel-filled implants that all bleed silicone continuously. What's more, in the rare instances that saline-filled implants do leak, it's only harmless saline—sterile saltwater in the same concentrations found naturally in blood—which the body simply absorbs.

Most doctors don't realize how vastly improved today's saline implants really are. Partly that's because the information U.S. makers include in each package still originate from outdated studies from the early 1970s of the earliest implants that suggest that the deflation rate may be as high as 76 percent. (One of those studies, in fact, was based on results with only 34 inflatable implants back in 1971!) That "disclosure" may well limit manufacturers' liability should a saline implant deflate, but it also unnecessarily undermines patients' and doctors' confidence in the product. No wonder many doctors seldom gave saline implants a chance.

But there's no excuse for the outright lies some doctors are telling patients, apparently to divert criticism away from themselves for having used the gel implants for so many years after their risks were suspected. For example, patients tell me that some plastic surgeons are saying the saline implants must be replaced every three to four years.

Wrong. If an implant fails at all, it usually happens within the first six months. And though that is undoubtedly upsetting, at least you know it's leaking. Unlike silicone implants that keep their shape even as they leach their contents, when a saline implant leaks, the breast slowly reverts back to its original size over a week's time. Afterward, the empty shell of solid silicone rubber—which, unlike the gel, contains no loose molecules to travel about the body—should be surgically removed and replaced. However, that can usually be done as a simple 20-minute office procedure under local anesthesia. Plastic surgeons aren't worried about untoward health effects from saline leakage; rather, they're afraid that they would find their busy practices disrupted with patients returning for replacement implants. Doctors much prefer dealing with silicone gel–filled implants. Patients don't have a clue when gel-filled implants leak or rupture, except perhaps when they come down with some vague complaint, such as swollen lymph nodes or a lump in their breasts.

How Do They Look?

Another fallacy that plastic surgeons cling to is the notion that the cosmetic result with saline-filled implants is not as good as with silicone gel–filled implants. This is simply not true. In my practice, saline implants have given superior results overall. The breasts stay softer and look better. That saline-filled implants produce the best result is not just my opinion; the reason they were first marketed was that study after study showed a far lower rate of tight, painful, disfiguring scar tissue capsules forming around them when compared with gel-filled implants. In my experience, the incidence of constrictive capsules is about 8 percent, compared with silicone gel–filled implants, which average nearly 75 percent. And, when tight capsules do form with saline-filled implants, they are not nearly as severe as with gel-filled implants.

Saline Requires Skill

Perhaps the plastic surgeons' biggest secret as to why they never used saline-filled implants is that they require more experience and skill in the operating room than silicone gel–filled implants. The latter go directly from the box into the patient because the silicone gel fill has been put in at the factory. Saline implants, however, arrive full of air. The surgeon must completely deflate each one in the operating room and then place it behind the breast before filling it with precisely the proper amount of saline. This also enables surgeons to customize each implant, as women's breasts are seldom exactly the same size.

It's an art, really. A tad too much saline, and the implant will feel too firm; too little, and it will wrinkle. Leave any air bubbles in the implant, and you can wind up with implants that slosh. The implants come in sizes according to how many cubic centimeters (cc's) of water they take. But because they are handmade, they can vary slightly in size. For example, if a surgeon takes an implant that is marked 240cc on its box and fills it with precisely that much water, some will be overfilled and feel quite firm; others will be underfilled and feel too loose and develop wrinkles. Only experience tells how much to fill the particular implant in order to get the best result.

Wrinkling causes a rippling effect that can be visible even when wearing a bra or bathing suit. It's a bigger problem for women who've undergone breast reconstruction after a mastectomy because they tend to have thinner skin covering the breast implant. It is rarely seen after augmentation. So, it is usually better to slightly overfill a reconstructive implant and to underfill a cosmetic one. Still, even plastic surgeons who do this every day can be fooled.

The correction of wrinkles consists of waiting a few months until the skin is completely relaxed and then reoperating under local anesthesia and injecting enough additional saline to balloon out the wrinkles. The best way is to sit the patient up while injecting the saline solution and watching the wrinkles disappear. The correction of overfilled implants naturally involves removing the excess. Again, one should wait several months. Unless a surgeon has become expert with saline implants, it's easy to see why so many eschewed them with the words, "Just get me one of those gel-filled implants off the shelf." Besides, since everyone else was using silicone, what could be wrong with them? Unfortunately, those were the words on their lips as they all went down to the sea like lemmings.

My Experience with Saline

I was introduced to saline-filled implants in the mid-1970s by a professor of plastic surgery on Long Island who had been using them for several months at his hospital. Not only did he rave about the improvement over the gel-filled implants but, more important, so did his resident staff. Resident surgeons are cynical and tell the truth. They see everything and nothing fazes them. After eight or ten years of constant decision making during hundred-hour workweeks relieved only by bad food and hard beds, resident surgeons tell it the way it is. They simply don't have the time or the temperament to tell it any other way.

I was impressed, so I started using the implants. Within a month or two, however, I was dismayed to learn from the professor that he had 45 saline implants deflate in his patients only months after they were placed. Now, this man, who has since died, was a very volatile person who lived as if the world was out to get him, and he viewed the leakages as further evidence of the world having once again singled him out for special punishment. He changed all the implants to silicone gel–filled ones and banned the use of saline-filled implants in his hospital.

The Root of the Problem

During the early days in the mid-1970s, I had a number of implants leak as well. But as I soon discovered, not all the problems with leakages were due to the implants. In fact, one cause was absolutely fascinating. The problem was that the body tissues adjacent to the saltwater implant's valve somehow sensed that there was a supply of water on the other side of the valve, and those tissues grew a root of pure collagen, which wormed its way through the valve and sucked out all the water. It was just like a plant that grows a root into a drainpipe to get water. If I had not seen the phenomenon personally, I would have found it quite unbelievable.

The tiny roots escaped surgeons' attention at first because they slipped out of the valve when the deflated implants were pulled out of their pockets behind the breast. But doctors became suspicious that something very unusual was going on when they later tested the deflated implants and found them to be perfectly intact. Their valves, too, were competent when tested. It was maddening until one day when a surgeon caught sight of the root and brought it to the attention of implant makers. Once he convinced them that this had indeed happened, the solution was simple. Implant makers designed a secondary plug that blocked the entrance to the valve. After that change, along with improvements in the manufacturing and quality control processes, leaks became relatively rare.

Different Models

Inevitably, plastic surgeons, who never like to leave anything as it is, put the basic, saline-filled bag through some changes. Of course, doctors who put a slightly different spin on a model put their name on it with the hope of perhaps getting a royalty on sales, promoting their practices, and being advanced in rank in their medical centers. Thus, we now have implants that come in "high-profile" or "low-profile" styles, in round or oval shapes, and with smooth or textured surfaces, each making its own claims as leading to more pleasing results. Though not all the various models that have come out are improvements, seductive claims made by

The Truth about Breast Implants

manufacturers are legion. In fact, they are typically made by the plastic surgeon who invented them, usually in a cooperative venture with the manufacturer. Implant makers think it is more effective to have a doctor as a front man when they're peddling products at their booths at national conventions.

It requires experience and a lot of acquired skepticism not to be taken in by the plausible but often specious claims. I recommend the smooth, round, low-profile implants with diaphragm valves. But a woman should be able to navigate her own way around the hype so that, in consultation with her doctor, she can pick the implant that's best for her. Here's a quick primer on the options:

- High vs. Low Profile. Low-profile implants are symmetrical; that is, they have the same curved shape in the front as in the back. The high profile, by contrast, has much more projection up front. It was developed in response to complaints by women who, after undergoing breast reconstruction, found that the front of their reconstructed breasts were round and flat and would not fit easily into a bra. However, from what I have learned, the high-profile design doesn't deliver for women with tight breast skin because the forward-protruding part of the high-profile implant becomes flattened. If the implant balloons backward, the front part becomes loose and can lead to wrinkles. At any rate, it seems to me that if the implant really could push the skin forward to a bra-fitting point, the risk would be that it might eventually push its way right through the skin. I prefer the symmetrical low-profile implants because their design distributes the fluid forces evenly, leading to fewer wrinkles and no risky pressure points.

- Round vs. Oval. The oval-shaped implant is also supposed to make the upper part of the breast jut out more
naturally and, like the high-profile variety, shares the
same drawbacks. Wrinkling may even be more severe
with the oval, I believe, because the saline does not
always adequately fill the top of the implant because of
gravity. Round implants, naturally, are less prone to
these potential problems because of the even distribu-
tion of fluid force against the implant.

- Smooth vs. Textured. Unfortunately, the textured-shell
implants are now all the rage in plastic surgery. In
theory, textured, like foam-covered implants, are supposed to trap scar tissue fibers as they form around the
implant so that they cannot lay down uniformly in parallel and tighten up. (See the discussion of polyurethane-covered implants in Chapter 1.) The only problem
is that the theory proved false 20 years ago in my
original studies at New York's Memorial Sloan-Kettering
Cancer Center, and it is false today. Textured-shell implants develop constrictive capsules just as often as
smooth-shell implants. For some reason, each new gen-
eration of surgeons has to find out for itself. Another
drawback is that textured implants must have thicker
shells, which make the implants unnaturally firm to
begin with. I always recommend smooth-shell implants;
they're much thinner and more elastic, and they make
for a more natural looking and feeling breast.

- Single- vs. Double-Compartment Implants. The so-
called double-lumen implant consists of an inner envelope filled with silicone gel surrounded by an outer
second shell filled with saline. These implants are now

subject to the same restrictions as single-lumen gel-filled implants. The marketing of these in the mid-1980s was a backhanded admission on the part of the implant's inventors that there was a serious problem with gel-filled implants. Its clever design allowed gel users to continue to use the implant without making a sudden leap to saline. As discussed in Chapter 1, proponents claimed that the double shell would substantially prevent the passage of silicone molecules out of the implant. Why this concept was ever taken seriously has always been a mystery. The simple truth is that any silicone molecule that will pass through one wall of these two-walled implants will eventually pass through the second. When confronted with this simple concept, the double-lumen users would reply that the second wall retarded the process. Even this is doubtful. When left for a short time, these implants develop a greasy feel and leave a telltale ring on a tabletop just like their single compartment cousins. Even if the passage of silicone were retarded by months, what difference would that make over a lifetime?

- Diaphragm vs. Leaf Valve. To be self-sealing, diaphragm valves are held closed by the elasticity of the surrounding plastic and must be forced open by a special tube for filling. They also come equipped with a strap closure that plugs up the valve opening—the design change made in the mid-1970s that keeps the body's collagen root out. By contrast, designers of leaf valves rely on positive pressure inside the implant to keep two internal leafs together, closing the valve. The only problem is that in the body, movement causes both positive and negative pressure phases inside the implant. The negative-pressure phase opens the valve slightly, allowing a small amount of saline to enter the leaf tunnel. A following positive phase pushes the saline along the tunnel. The amounts are small, but the numerous positive-to-negative pressure swings eventually may deflate the implant. In my experience, these implants do leak, and I recommend very strongly that one use an implant with a diaphragm valve.

Saline Goes under the FDA Microscope

A good deal of scientific evidence on precisely which design features work best is likely to emerge now that safety and effectiveness studies of saline-filled implants are going to the FDA. The FDA, acting on a legislative mandate to begin reviewing over 160 medical devices (basically any medical product that is not a drug) is expected to review the studies by sometime in 1994. Because these implants are filled with harmless saline and a solid silicone rubber shell, no one expects the kind of media circus that hearings on silicone gel–filled implants turned into. For one thing, of course, saline implants contain no silicone gel or liquid. What's more, though the envelope that holds the saltwater is made of solid silicone, it is thin enough, and saltwater is transparent enough, that X rays can more easily pass through, meaning that saline implants don't interfere as much with mammography. (See Chapter 6.)

Until all the data in support of the safety and efficacy of saline implants are in, it's a good idea for women considering breast reconstruction and augmentation to discuss the risks with a doctor who is knowledgeable about saline-filled implants. (See the discussion of how to find a surgeon in Chapter 2.) Compared with silicone gel–filled implants, the risks of using saline implants—such as infection, leakage, firmness, improper position, and wrinkling—come more under the heading of nuisances than of serious problems. They occur quite rarely and are usually correctable. With saline-filled implants, if the whole experience turns bad, the implant can be removed, and, except for a minimal scar where the implant was put in, the patient will be where she started with no harm being done. The most ancient adage of surgery, *primum non nocere* (first, do no harm), has been upheld.

Risk of Infection

Infection with saline-filled implants is very rare: less than one in a thousand cases in large studies. Studies show that the most commonly isolated cause is the *Staphylococcus epidermis* bacterium, a common skin contaminant. It's not a life-threatening complication (none of the risks of saline implants are), but still no one likes nasty infections that are sometimes difficult to get rid of. In those rare instances when it does happen, the patient typically returns to the doctor's office several days after implantation complaining of a low fever and a red, swollen breast. Normally, the patient is put on antibiotics and told to record her temperature twice a day: once in the morning, when it should be lowest, and once in the late afternoon, when temperatures are normally at their highest. Sometimes weeks go by and patients still have temperatures of about 100 or so; some days they don't have fevers at all, but the breast stays swollen. The redness may even disappear.

But if there's an infection, a woman can nearly always tell that there's something not quite right. If an infection is present, after three to five weeks the temperature will climb unmistakably, and the breast will become hard and tender to the touch. And at that point, with symptoms worsening, the implant really has to come out because the body can't get rid of the infection with the implant in the way. Typically, a few days after the removal, the symptoms subside. But the implant cannot be replaced for about four months, a situation no one likes very much. This can happen just as easily in cosmetic as in reconstructive cases. If it happens to you, try not to lose faith in your surgeon. Infections are sometimes not explainable, like acts of God. Try to be patient while the implant is out. It will look just as well in the end. I have never had a patient become infected twice in a row.

What about Leaking?

As stated earlier in this chapter, leakage of implants is rare, being in the range of 1 in 300 or 400. Leaks virtually always are traced to a manufacturing defect that could not be found by quality control testing. When the defect is in the shell, the problem may be a thin spot or an error in the envelope's crossweave that leaves a tiny hole that scarcely allows even a dribble of water to pass through when the implant is squeezed. If the shell has no hole and the implant is deflated, one can only surmise that the valve is defective. I squeeze and massage each implant thoroughly before inserting it to try to find defects. Unfortunately, some show up only later.

It's good advice for all women who get implants to ask for the name of the implant, its identification number, and the manufacturer and to keep them with their medical records in case there ever is a problem. Since August of 1993, your surgeon is, by law, required to give you this information. You should also consider signing up with an implant registry such as the one offered by the Medic-Alert group (see Appendix). This organization will automatically contact you if a problem with your type of implant ever arises. (For information, call [800] 892-9211.) Still, because leakage usually happens within the first few months after implantation, I tell patients who experience no problem after the first six months that their chances of experiencing a problem in the future are extremely small.

Rupturing

Of course, it is possible for an implant actually to rupture if the trauma is severe enough, say, in a blow from a steering wheel during an automobile accident. Lesser impact from athletics, hugging, or active sex do not break saline implants. Even if an actual rupture does occur, the implant still does not suddenly deflate. The water remains in the tissue pocket containing the implant until it is absorbed by the body. This can take days. If the implant leaks, it does not mean that the original surgery needs to be done all over again. Most of the time spent at the original operation was in the making of the space under the skin or the breast to hold the implant. Reopening the entrance to this space and changing one implant for another is quite simple and can be done under local anesthesia in about 20 minutes.

Hardening

After leakage, hardening of the implants is probably a patient's biggest concern. Actually, it is not the implants but the capsule of scar tissue that surrounds them that becomes firm. They can constrict implants and make the breasts feel hard and painful. Unfortunately, it is not possible to predict who will form a tight, thick capsule and who will not. The overall incidence with saline-filled implants is in the range of eight to ten percent as compared with that of the gel-filled implants, which in large studies show an average incidence many times as high.

Because there is no liquid silicone in saline-filled implants, the only known cause of tight capsule formation is blood clotting around the implant. If even a small amount of blood oozes from the raw pocket walls after implantation, this will clot around the implant, making it feel hard right away. In addition, the clotting provides a matrix into which scar tissue will grow to make it feel harder yet. Most doctors use three tactics to combat capsules. First, surgical drainage tubes are used to suck out any blood that accumulates after the wound is closed. These are left in place for 24 hours. Second, elastic bandages are wrapped around the chest to compress the implant and its pocket to reduce the chance of interior bleeding.

The Truth about Breast Implants

The third tactic adds a small amount of a natural steroid (called cortisone) to the saline in the implant. In large doses, cortisone can thin the skin, which is why I use a very small amount—less than the body makes on its own in a day. The cortisone leaches out of the implant over a period of four to six weeks, bathing the surface of the implant. Cortisone interferes with the transport of collagen (the basic constituent of scar tissue), which is made by special cells called fibroblasts. This reduces the volume of scar tissue produced. Cortisone also causes the fibroblast to make defective collagen fibers that cannot bond together and thus cannot shrink to tighten firmly around an implant. The incidence of tight capsule formation is much lower now than it was before the use of cortisone.

If a very tight capsule does form, an operation is sometimes necessary. The surgeon reenters the pocket behind the breast, using the same point of entry as the first time so that there is not a second scar, and cuts through the scar capsule from the inside, slicing it into disjointed sections. When this is finished, the capsule looks a bit like a peeled banana skin with its sections splayed apart. If done thoroughly, the capsule that reforms usually does not tighten up again. However, it is only fair to say that there are some people, probably only about two to four percent, who are prone to form capsules, and they will form a tight capsule no matter how many times they have the procedure. The same small number will experience a loss of sensation in the nipple or develop an area of numbness, usually on the lower half of the breast, that is often temporary but can be permanent after cosmetic enlargement.

Too High or Too Low

Of the lesser complications attributable to saline implants, the most common is that the implant is not in the correct position. It's too high, too low, too much toward the middle, too much toward the side. If this is discovered right after surgery, the implant can simply be positioned correctly by manipulating it into place and holding it there for a week with a specially padded bra (that is, provided that the surgically created pocket behind the breast was made in the right spot at surgery).

However, position problems can show up after a few weeks, when the swelling and tightness of the chest has passed. The problem is still correctable, but another operation may be necessary. Though it is usually a minor procedure, often done under local anesthesia, patients have to go back to the hospital for a couple of hours. Fortunately, this is rare.

Similarly, sometimes after mastectomy reconstructions, tight breast tissues stretch too much, making the implant appear a bit large. Or tissue that's too tight can make the implant look too small. The solution, of course, is to replace the implant. Even in simple breast enlargement, when the swelling from surgery subsides, the breasts can look too big or too small. Changing the implant without further charge has to be part of the deal from the beginning. After all, a woman cannot be absolutely sure what size she wants until she has had a chance to live with the new breasts for a month or two.

6

⤬

After Implantation

Getting on with
Your Life

Saline-filled implants allow women to get on with their lives without the worry about liquid silicone permeating their bodies. There's no need for frequent return visits to the doctor's office that women with silicone gel–filled implants are often asked to make—and for good reason. The growing list of suspected problems for which women with silicone gel must keep ever vigilant simply does not apply to saline users. I tell my patients to return for follow-up visits after six months or a year, unless they have any problems, of course. Most women really don't need any more follow-up visits than that.

Women who've undergone breast reconstruction obviously must see their cancer surgeons as often as he or she feels necessary for treatment and to monitor for recurrence. But for women who have simple cosmetic breast enlargements with saline-filled implants, there isn't anything that a plastic surgeon would see that wouldn't be perfectly obvious to patients themselves. And more important, the things that can go wrong aren't terribly serious. For instance, in the rare occasion that a saline-filled implant deflates, the patient will be aware of it. The same is true if at some point the implant looks like it is in the wrong spot. And if it gets hard, she'll know that, too. Obviously, if these problems arise, women should go immediately back to their plastic surgeon.

The First Three Weeks after Enlargement

The breasts require no special care. There is really not much you can do to make them better or worse. Typically, for the first three weeks, women simply are restricted from doing anything that would raise their blood pressure or bounce their breasts around, such as jogging, playing tennis, playing golf, lifting heavy suitcases, or going to exercise class. The reason for the three-week period is that the surgically made pocket that holds the implant behind the breast needs time to heal. It is during those first three weeks that the area is most susceptible to bleeding, which is the prime cause of tight capsule formation and firm to hard results. But women can do normal things right away, such as drive a car, push a cart in a market, reach up into shelves, go for long walks, and go back to work. And after three weeks they can do absolutely anything.

I always advise my patients not to go straight from the operating room to Victoria's Secret and spend a lot of money on new bras, at least until the normal postoperative swelling goes down within the first few weeks of surgery. Otherwise, the bras might be too large later on. A cotton sport bra works just fine because it comes in small, medium, and large sizes and is most comfortable during that time.

The First Few Months after Reconstruction

For women after breast reconstruction, there's no need to wear any support at all during the first few months because the reconstructed side is initially flattened and firm. The goal is to get the reconstructed breast to droop as much as possible. Over this time, the soft tissues of the breast will stretch, and the breast will become softer, more prominent, and slightly pendulous. I don't believe that anyone has ever developed a one-sided jogging bra, but that would be the ideal support to wear.

Of course, if a woman thinks her reconstructed breast is getting too droopy, she should see her plastic surgeon. The same is true if new scar tissue pushes or pulls the implant out of position. Sometimes the doctor can provide a specially padded bra that can put pressure on the implant so that it settles down into its proper position. In rare cases, adjustment surgery may be necessary after about three months, at which point the implant has pretty much settled in place. At this time the doctor might open up the pocket behind the breast to let the implant drop a bit more or raise the implant by closing up the space where it's not wanted. This is also the time a woman might consider having her natural breast adjusted somewhat—either reduced, enlarged, or lifted—to help attain the best possible symmetry. Nipple reconstruction, if desired, would best start now, too. (See Chapter 3.)

The First Year after Tissue Transplantation

There is a bizarre and fairly common side effect women should watch for after undergoing back-muscle (latissimus dorsi) transfers. For six months to a year, they're liable to find that the transplanted back muscle that now covers the breast twitches. The reason is that the brain's movement centers take many months to adapt to the fact that the muscle that was in back is now in front and that the former back muscle should no longer be activated for back movements. It's confusing for the brain. Until the brain catches on, the breast can really jump around, which can lead to some embarrassing situations, as you might imagine. Unfortunately, nothing can be done to prevent this. It's just a matter of time but usually no more than 12 months until the brain adapts itself to this new situation.

An important precaution after breast reconstruction is to avoid a bad sunburn. The skin covering a reconstructed breast after a mastectomy is thin, and the blood supply is diminished. Most people don't realize that the blood supply of the body is not only its heating mechanism but also its cooling mechanism. If the skin is heated by sunlight, the blood flow normally takes the heat away. But if the blood supply is diminished and cannot take the heat away at a normal rate, then the heat builds up in the tissues and actually cooks them. I had one patient who had a peekaboo bathing-suit top. It had a series of holes that started up around the shoulder and got smaller as they approached the center of the breast. But the sun was able to hit the skin at full strength through these holes. At the smallest, which was about the size of a dime, there was a circular burn straight through the skin. The implant had to be removed until the skin healed.

The Massage Myth

Doctors very often tell their patients to massage their breasts after implantation. The theory is that by pushing the implant around, a woman can maintain a larger sized pocket and keep the implant loose and, therefore, soft. Unfortunately, massage often pushes implants out of position. It's simple anatomy. The tissues tend to be tighter at the bottom of the chest than at the top. (Feel your own chest. You can grab a bunch of skin under your collarbone and move it around, but you can't do that quite so well down around the ribs because it is tighter at the bottom.) So, if you keep moving the implant around, the implant keeps getting stepped up as the loose skin relaxes at the top and the tight skin closes at the bottom. And high implants produce bulges at the top of the breast, which is a dead giveaway that you have a breast implant.

Doctors who prescribe daily massage say that it's important because it helps stretch the scar tissue that encases the implant. Aside from pushing the implant out of position, the scar tissue responds to the challenge by getting thicker and tighter, not softer. Nature, in our jungle days, gave us scar tissue to help us heal as quickly and as solidly as possible before the tiger tracked us down and ate us. Nature won't easily let anything defeat its purpose. That is why scars around joints and wherever there's movement are always heavier. Just look at the wide, heavy scars of people who've had knee or elbow operations. So if you massage the pocket, the movement is going to produce heavier scar tissue. And that, in addition to pushing the implant around and making it end up in the wrong spot, may also constrict it and make it feel hard.

There's even some concern that massage might weaken implants, according to findings of a recent congressional subcommittee staff report. Though the report deals with gel-filled, not saline-filled, implants, one concern raised about massage may be equally applicable. The report cited a February 1984 memorandum from Eldon Frisch, a Dow Corning scientist, who was worried that the breast exercises many plastic surgeons were instructing patients to do could cause progressive weakening of the implants and ultimately rupture. (Frisch also hypothesized that the exercises could cause the gel in silicone gel–filled implants to break down, making it less cohesive, a worry that happily does not apply to saline users.) As the report states, there is no evidence that this memo was made available to plastic surgeons right up to the point that it was handed over to government investigators in February 1992.

Saline Implants and Mammography

Breast cancer detection is important for all women, including those who undergo augmentation and reconstruction. Women who have had their breasts rebuilt after cancer might find it helpful to speak plainly with their oncologists about how often they should get mammograms, or breast X rays, of the remaining breast, along with physician checkups and self-examinations. There's no reason to have X rays on the mastectomized side because no breast tissue remains after a mastectomy. Women who have simple cosmetic enlargements might wish to speak with their doctors about the advisability of getting mammograms before surgery.

The American College of Radiology (ACR) recommends that all women over the age of 35 have "baseline" breast X rays taken before surgery to detect unsuspected cancer and to serve as a comparison against future mammograms because change is one of the most important things the radiologist looks for. Afterward, most women would do well to follow the American Cancer Society's recommendations. That is, by age 40, women without symptoms should have mammographic screenings performed every one to two years. Beginning at age 50, the guidelines state, mammography should be performed annually. (A physical examination of the breast by a doctor is also recommended every three years for women 20 to 40 and every year for those over 40.) Studies suggest that whether a woman has an implant or not, mammography is the key to early diagnosis of breast cancer because it can help detect the tiniest tumors when they are most treatable.

For women with implants, it's best to ask for a referral to an American College of Radiology–approved mammography center that has technicians with expertise in taking X rays of women with implants. You may wish to call the ACR at (800) 227-6440 to find out if a given facility is accredited. In addition, the American Cancer Society ([800] ACS-2345) and the National Cancer Institute ([800] 4-CANCER) will help steer women to accredited centers in their areas.

The Truth about Breast Implants

All implants partially block X rays, obscuring breast tissue that otherwise could be analyzed for signs of tumors. But most experts agree that saline-filled implants don't cast as heavy a shadow on X ray film as silicone gel–filled implants. What's more, mammographers expert in taking X rays of women with implants can use a special technique to minimize the interference by temporarily pushing the implant out of the X ray beam's field. The technique, called the Eklund method after the doctor who developed it, involves gently pushing the implant back against the chest wall while pulling the breast tissue over and in front of it for a few seconds before mammogram views are taken. It's a technique that takes experience and skill to perform. So, if your mammographer seems clumsy in the technique, I'd suggest you insist on waiting for a better trained technician or else seek an appointment elsewhere.

According to the American College of Radiology, although there are currently no controlled trials demonstrating reduced effectiveness of early detection with mammography in women with breast implants, those contemplating augmentation should be informed that mammography may be more difficult to perform, and it may be less effective. Recently, a report in the *Journal of the American Medical Association* on women with silicone gel–filled implants suggested that the main culprit in obscuring breast X rays is capsular contracture: the condition characterized by tightening and hardening of the scar tissue that surrounds an implant. The reason the capsules interfered was that they made it difficult for mammographers to perform the Eklund maneuver and flatten the breast against the plates in the mammography machine. Women with the most severe contractures came out with almost completely unreadable X rays showing only a thin corona of breast tissue around the shadow cast by the implant. Because saline-filled implants have far lower rates of capsular contracture, this study seems to attest to saline's superiority. However, women should also know that the capsules can interfere in another way. If mineral salts become deposited in the capsule (what's known as calcification), it can compromise breast X rays and lead to diagnostic errors.

In the past, there was another type of mammogram, called a xerogram, which in some studies produced virtually unobscured breast X rays right through saline-filled implants. The problem was that it delivered far too much radiation, and today its use in clinical mammography programs has all but disappeared. Ultrasound, which uses high-frequency waves instead of radiation to image breast tissue, readily penetrates breast implants but cannot detect some of the earliest and tiniest indicators of cancer. Though it is too expensive and time consuming to use as a screen, ultrasound is worthwhile in following up suspicious mammograms. It can differentiate benign cysts from possibly malignant solid masses, which should be examined further or biopsied, something mammography alone cannot do.

Getting on with Your Life

In weighing the risks of breast implants and discussing what can go wrong, it's important not to lose sight of the profound psychological benefits saline-filled implants can have both for cancer patients trying to cope with the scars of cancer surgery and for healthy women who wish merely to

The Truth about Breast Implants

have larger breasts. They discover their self-confidence and feel more attractive, feminine, and desirable. Of course, those few who are pursuing careers as models or actresses delight in the possibility that their careers may be enhanced. But the vast majority of women are happy just to be able to go out to a dinner party and wear a relatively low cut dress and show cleavage. Those who have lost a breast to cancer surgery are usually thrilled simply to be able to look natural in a bathing suit. Many have confided that they feel as if they'd become a whole person again. It's a phrase I've heard many times: "a whole person." To others, it was as if they had been in a boxing match with the odds against them and come out the victor. Going through breast reconstruction, one patient told me, was her badge, her proof that she had overcome cancer.

Here, in their own words, are the stories of two women whose lives changed dramatically for the better. The first, a New York businesswoman named Dolores Broad, was one of the first women in the country to undergo breast reconstruction. Because it was 1971, a silicone gel–filled implant was used; I replaced it with a saline-filled implant soon after they came on the market. Reconstruction so changed her life that she went around the country spreading the word. She started self-help groups for women and counseled them before and after their reconstructions. Here is Dolly's story:

"As a young woman in my 30s, discovering that I had a breast tumor and had to have a mastectomy came as a very big shock. I was emotionally devastated by my surgery. The only way to explain it is ... destruction. Of course, I was thankful that I was alive but I more hated what I was left with.

"My husband kept trying to reassure me that I was still a very lovely lady and that I was still desirable ... that all the qualities that had made him fall in love with me were still there. But I felt like I no longer loved myself. Because of that it was a very difficult time in our marriage. I would not go to bed with him unless I was all covered up.

"I felt my surgery had made a lesser woman of me, not only sexually—but of me. I felt like a different person. I felt all out of balance. You know you have two arms, two legs, women have two breasts. And if you're missing an arm or a leg you become unbalanced and deformed and that's how I felt—deformed, unbalanced and ugly. When I first had my surgery I felt as though God had punished me for something terrible that I had done. It made me depressed and remorseful.

"The mastectomy had been done in February so I could wear turtlenecks and things that covered everything when I went out. But then April and May came and I started thinking about summer. How was I going to walk around New York in the heat? I started hounding my surgeon. Something has to be done, I told him. If you can't I'll go and find somebody to do something. He introduced me to Dr. Guthrie.

"At that time he was just researching breast reconstruction. Dow Corning was making the only implants and they were available in three sizes: small, medium and large. He told me what the surgery would involve and said, 'I'm willing to take a chance if you are.' I was.

"He did my reconstruction in September 1971. It made me feel . . . like I had regained my balance. It made me feel so much better about myself and about my relationships with other people. Afterward, my husband said he couldn't believe how much difference this made in me. For months, I had been quiet and withdrawn thinking that maybe this isn't the best way to spend a life. And then after the reconstruction, I became myself again. I became this flag-bearer for

The Truth about Breast Implants

reconstruction giving programs and talking before groups. It's been over 20 years ... now I don't even think about it anymore. I'm fine now and when I look in the mirror, I still look pretty good."

Simple breast enlargement with saline-filled implants also helped this next woman blossom. This woman, who lives in the Midwest, is not my patient. But there are women everywhere who have shared her feelings. To protect her privacy, I'll call her Susan. Here is her story, in her own words:

"I was never comfortable with my body because I always had very small breasts. Even in my 20s I used to buy my bras in the children's department. I was around a double-A cup, which is pretty much nothing. My husband always told me he was very happy with the way I was and I suppose that was enough for me. But when I got older and had a child and nursed for 14 months my breasts just lost their life, they were no longer even acceptable to me. I don't think that my husband found me all that attractive, though he never said anything about it. I think that there was a period of about five years where I really seriously considered having implants before going through with it.

"I know that to someone who isn't in this situation, getting implants can sound very foolish but you have to understand that when you're so uncomfortable in clothes or out of clothes it makes you very unhappy. I realized that it wasn't going to change my life in terms of the quality of what kind of person I am. But I felt it was going to make me feel better about me.

"I was pear-shaped. I had a hippy figure—I'm not now.... I'm well proportioned because now I have breasts but before I felt like I was all bottom. I was even very narrow through my rib cage. So clothes never looked right, even just wearing a dress. And I found that if I wore separates in bathing suits, it was especially embarrassing. I never could go out on a boat with a group of people and feel comfortable— you know, any situation where you are obvious and compared to other women. I think that, more than anything else, really bothered me.

"I just knew that my breast size was something that could be changed about me. It was almost like a fantasy. I wouldn't have to envy someone for their physical attributes or wish I was someone else.

"It was in the summer three years ago that I finally had implants filled with saline put in. When I buy bras now they're B-cups. I wanted to be very tasteful, I didn't want to be bosomy, I didn't want to be called booby. It was nothing sexual. I just wanted breasts like a normal woman. I wanted just to be able to wear clothes and feel comfortable with myself.

"Now I'm perfectly happy being me. I'm now divorced—so it's true that having a perfect figure doesn't really make for a perfect life. But I wouldn't change anything. I'll tell you that I listen to my body more now but I haven't regretted one minute. And I have friends look at me and say enviously, 'You're disgusting, they're perfect.' And they are perfect because I had something done to them to make them that way and they're still very, very nice."

Those stories typify the experiences of women with the best results. Of course, saline-filled implants do not solve all of life's problems, but they can help people close the door on an unpleasant chapter in their lives and begin anew. That's something no one can yet say with certainty about silicone gel–filled implants.

EPILOGUE

୧୨

Putting It All in Perspective

The Decline of Ethics and the Need for Responsibility

Now that we've come to the end of this book, there are three important messages I would like to leave with you. The first is that saline-filled implants are safe and must not be confused with silicone gel–filled implants, which are not safe. The FDA's review will undoubtedly lead to that conclusion. The second is that even if gel-filled implants were safe, saline-filled implants would still be preferable because they give better cosmetic results. And the third is that rebuilding a breast with a saline-filled implant is far safer than with any sort of tissue transplant. The common denominator of all those messages is this: If you have to have a breast procedure and your doctor does not offer you a saline-filled implant as an option, seek another opinion; resorting to anything else will most likely leave you so sorry and anguished later on that you may well wish that you had done nothing at all.

You may say, "Well, if that's the message and it's so simple, why is there all this controversy?" The answer is that the plastic surgeon community got itself started with gel-filled implants. As you learned in Chapter 1, when implants first came out 30 years ago, they were such a dramatic improvement over anything that existed before that their use became universal almost overnight. Some problems were detected early, such as hardening, but these were things that everyone was willing to live with. Realization of the silicone bleed phenomenon came slowly and at a time during the 1970s when there was no alternative to the gel-filled implant. To the vast majority of plastic surgeons, it did not seem serious enough to warrant stopping breast enlargement altogether. Of course, by this time, the procedure had also become the number one money maker in plastic surgery.

When the alternative of saline-filled implants became available, many of the early models were defective and leaked. Although they leaked only saltwater, which was absorbed by the body with no harmful effects, the breast noticeably deflated after a few days. Most plastic surgeons used that as an excuse to not even take the time to learn the technique. Implanting saline-filled implants is, after all, more demanding because they must be filled with just the right amount of saltwater by surgeons during implantation. By the time the saline-filled implants' leaking problem was solved, plastic surgeons had already made up their minds. Most refused to accept that the improvements were true or satisfactory. It was easier simply to claim that saline-filled implants still leaked or still wrinkled and to continue using silicone gel–filled implants. At least if the gel-filled implants leaked, many plastic surgeons felt at the time, it wouldn't be immediately noticeable.

Until today, no one wanted to focus on the problem of the dissemination of liquid silicone into the body. It was convenient to assume that this was not a problem. As far as anyone knew, silicone was inert.

The Attitude Problem

Plastic surgeons were not always so unquestioning. A little over 40 years ago, plastic surgery was still a small fraternity of about 500 general surgeons who had chosen to specialize in this new field. Among them were some of the giants of surgery. They existed only in the main medical centers and were under the supervision of the chiefs of general surgery, who would never have tolerated the shenanigans of today. Those were more serious times, and medicine in all fields was much more rigorously controlled both in training and in practice.

Sometime in the mid-1960s, plastic surgery began to break away from general surgery. Many fewer plastic surgeons completed a full residency in general surgery; fewer became certified by the American Board of Surgery before entering plastic surgery. Many rejected the tradition of earlier years, during which time a period of full-time service in a teaching hospital, including time spent in charity clinics and the laboratories, was a prerequisite to gaining university hospital privileges after finishing residency training. This way to success had promised little immediate monetary reward but

The Truth about Breast Implants

offered the chance to develop experience and reputation that would slowly lead to referrals from the older, established doctors in the medical center. It also led to promotion in academic rank. Being appointed an instructor in a medical school was a major event. Eventually, the best would move up through the ranks to become assistant professor, associate professor, and, if the gods were with them, full professor.

But with cosmetic surgery blossoming during the 1960s and the incomes of plastic surgeons doubling and tripling, young doctors were becoming anxious to establish their private practices as soon as possible in order to reap their rewards. The cost of education had increased dramatically, and many plastic surgeons finishing their training had accumulated staggering debts. The field became more freewheeling. The decade of the 1960s had taught the young that they did not have to sacrifice to get what they wanted. They could find shortcuts, and so they did. One could circumvent having to put in the years of work to earn the respect of one's peers.

A relative pittance paid to a public relations firm could get one's name touted before the public as a major figure in the medical world. Why did one need referrals from doctors when one television appearance or one magazine article could bring the world to one's door? I trained a plastic surgeon who, a month after finishing his residency, was on national television as the foremost expert in the country in the field of breast reconstruction. I knew that he had not yet done a single case on his own.

Who needed academic rank, many young doctors thought to themselves, when one could make millions without it? The medical schools were the last sanctuaries of the old ethics, and they demanded that doctors do their part in the clinics caring for poor people. Advertising and the use of public relations were anathema. The medical schools believed that you could not maintain quality unless you enforced standards that encouraged an orderly progression of learning and skill. The problem was that the young had decided that the standards required too many years and too much work. If they didn't get the academic rank—and that is the one thing that they never have gotten—money and fame were more than a good trade.

The number of training programs increased dramatically. And there was no dearth of applicants for what was increasingly being perceived as the gold mine of all medical specialties. The result was a rapid overpopulation of plastic surgeons, which made earning a living more competitive and the commercial side of the profession much too important. In fact, it was getting harder every day to think of plastic surgery as a profession in the old sense.

Falling Standards

In the mid-1970s, the courts decided that doctors could sue hospitals that would not give them privileges or tried to discipline them. The ethics committees of the county medical societies—which had been the upholders of standards in America for 200 years and were the inheritors of the guilds who had done the same since the days of ancient Egypt—suddenly were the victims of disgruntled, usually substandard doctors whom the committees had had to discipline. We entered the age of litigation, with every lawyer getting a third of the judgments according to the contingency fee system tolerated in no other country on earth. The lower elements of medicine (and there are always lower elements in any sphere of life) were now out from under the control of their local peers, who were the only ones with the expertise to know them for what they were, and were now subject only to courts whose ignorance, incompetence, and ineffectiveness must be synonymous with the American 20th century.

Only the recognized specialty societies remained as upholders of standards. To be certified by the American Board of Plastic Surgery, a doctor had to be recommended by an approved training program and pass strenuous written and oral examinations given a year apart. This had been the backbone of guaranteeing high specialty standards for generations in the United States and was the envy of the world. But that backbone broke in the early 1980s, when the Federal Trade Commission brought suit against the specialty boards for restraint of trade. Suddenly, the boards were labeled monopolies and faced antitrust violations for upholding standards, approving only surgeons who trained in approved programs or who passed standard examinations given impartially to everyone.

At that time, the FDA had decided to leave the supervision of medical devices to doctors and essentially let the companies who made the devices understand that they could make anything that the doctors approved. Of course, if it was clear that the device was dangerous, the company would have liability, but if the doctors who were putting these devices into people every day in a huge human experiment did not think they were dangerous, why would the company even begin to think so? The manufacturers were simply in it for the money. Most of them had no idea of what they were making or doing. Their studies were incomplete, inadequate, sloppy, and poorly motivated.

At this point, not only had all constraints on standards been removed, but many of the old guard, who on other days could have been counted on to keep things under control, now had been attacked too often and threw up their hands and abandoned the struggle. The barbarians were not just at the gate, but they had already trampled it down. People were now going into plastic surgery with no effective control by hospitals, medical schools, county medical societies, specialty boards or their elders in the profession. The draw and the goal was only fame and money to be acquired overnight by promoting "new" medical devices on the latest evening talk show. Not having learned discipline, morals, ethics, or standards in their training programs, do you wonder that some of these people didn't give a fig about disseminating liquid silicone into your body? Do you really think that they would take time away from their money practice and do the extra work to learn a new procedure just because someone said that fluid silicone in the body might one day be a problem?

When I warned colleagues that this day was inevitable, they would say, "We don't know enough to change anything," and I would reply, "You know all you need to know. When the public knows as much as you know now, they are going to be outraged." That is, of course, exactly what has happened.

Take Charge

My goal in writing this book has been to tell you that the important truth about breast implants is that there is a bright side. With all the bad publicity about silicone implants—

which never mention that it's what's inside the implants that is important—you, like most women, may have been under the impression that all implants were bad, that there were no other options. In fact, many women still do not realize that saline-filled implants even exist. But saline-filled implants have long been available and are safe and viable for you, whether you wish to enlarge your breasts because you feel they're too small or to reclaim what cancer surgery has taken from you. Use what you've learned in this book to demand responsible medical care, and my work on this book will have been worthwhile. I wish you well.

APPENDIX

Contacts for Additional Information

All organizations below provide information about breast implants. However, these days it's impossible to vouch for the quality of information consumers will receive. For instance, former implant manufacturer Dow Corning still furnishes consumer information even though in 1991 it was caught giving out inaccurate information, according to the FDA. One FDA official who called Dow's 800 telephone hot-line pretended to be a college student and was told by Dow that implants are "100 percent safe." Misinformation like that earned the company an FDA warning letter.

Even the FDA's Breast Implant Information Service raises some questions, not about the information it provides but about confidentiality. If you order free information via the FDA's hotline number ([800] 532-4440), you will get a packet that includes a form that reads, "Individuals who request written information from the Breast Implant Information Line were included on a confidential mailing list. If you do not wish to receive any additional mailing from the FDA please

The Truth about Breast Implants

return this notice containing your extra mailing label within two weeks. . . . "

You will also notice that the American Society of Plastic and Reconstructive Surgeons, the major professional organization of plastic surgeons, is listed, even though its public information brochure *Straight Talk* . . . *About Breast Implants*, published in 1990, contains many glaring inaccuracies, as noted in Chapter 4. For instance, the brochure claims that capsular contracture affects "one out of ten women," whereas the research literature at the time reported 30 to 40 percent contracture rates. As always, the warning "buyer beware" applies.

Contacts for Additional Information

American Cancer Society

1599 Clifton Road, NE

Atlanta, GA 30329

For local offices call: (800) ACS-2345

> Local offices provide written information on implants and breast reconstruction as well as over 2,000 other subjects. Information is updated monthly. The ACS's in-hospital Reach to Recovery program pairs mastectomy patients with volunteers for information and support.

American Society of Plastic and Reconstructive Surgeons

444 East Algonquin Road

Arlington Heights, IL 60005

(800) 635-0635

> This professional medical society of about 5,000 plastic surgeons runs a 24-hour toll-free hotline that enables you to (1) check whether a plastic surgeon is board certified by the American Board of Plastic Surgery, (2) receive the names of five board-certified plastic surgeons in your area, (3) order brochures on plastic surgery procedures, and (4) ask specific medical questions of registered nurses on duty Monday through Friday from 8:30 A.M. to 4:30 P.M. (If appropriate, nurses may schedule a free telephone consultation or office-visit consultation with a plastic surgeon in your area.)

AS-IS (American Silicone Implant Survivors)
1288 Cork Elm Drive
Kirkwood, MO 63122
(314) 821-0115

Founded in 1990 by a woman who had suffered complications after various types of silicone gel–filled breast
implants, this group brings implant support-group lead-
ers together in national women's conferences, sponsors
annual symposia for medical professionals, and pre-
sents educational seminars for the general public. It
provides information researched by an advisory board of
medical professionals (packets of information cost $8 to
$25). The group makes referrals to medical practitioners
familiar with the problems of women with implants. Its
periodic newsletter costs $25 a year.

Boston Women's Health Book Collective
P.O. Box 192
Summerville, MA 02144
(617) 625-0271

This nonprofit group is an advocacy and information
center that collaborates with other organizations on
women's issues and reproductive health. It provides an
information package for a $10 donation that includes a
wide range of news and magazine clippings, information
on associated health issues, testimony from congressional hearings, and implant manufacturer–supplied information on implants.

Contacts for Additional Information

Breast Implant Information Foundation

P.O. Box 2907

Laguna Hills, CA 92654

(714) 448-9928

A nonprofit group begun by a woman who experienced medical complications from a variety of silicone gel–filled breast implants, this group provides $40 information packets that include medical journal citations, news accounts and papers on the components of silicone, and brief explanations about how they affect the body. Its monthly newsletter costs $25 a year; videotapes of guest speakers cost from $20 to $40.

Command Trust Network

For augmentation:

c/o Kathleen Anneken

P.O. Box 17082

Covington, KY 41017

For reconstruction:

c/o Sybil Goldrich

256 South Linden Drive

Beverly Hills, CA 90212

Founded by women who experienced complications after various silicone gel–filled breast implants, this group advocates further implant studies and provides information to consumers and professionals. Its information packet contains a newsletter, names of pathologists, and other helpful notices. To receive the packet, send a $2 check and a self-addressed stamped envelope. To receive its newsletter on a quarterly basis, send $15 a year.

Dow Corning
P.O. Box 994
Midland, MI 448686
(800) 442-5442

Once the largest implant manufacturer, this corporation answers questions about implants and will send an information packet about silicone gel–filled breast implants, including patient information booklets and information from the FDA. On request, it will send documents and scientific studies that have been released to the FDA. It will also send information about its implant-removal assistance program.

FDA Breast Implant Information Service
Consumer Affairs (HFE-88)
5600 Fishers Lane
Rockville, MD 20857
Hotline: (800) 532-4440

The FDA offers helpful information in summaries called "Talk Papers" as well as consumer pamphlets and resources. The FDA hotline provides recorded announcements on the latest information on FDA rulings concerning implants and allows callers to order the information package as well as forms that women can send in to describe any problems they might have experienced with implants.

Contacts for Additional Information

International Breast Implant Registry

2323 Colorado Avenue

Department 95X

Turlock, CA 95382

(800) 892-9211

This service was established by the nonprofit Medic Alert Foundation to track patients with implants and to locate and notify them—through their physicians and hospitals—in the event of a product recall or other important news about the device. This patient care service involves a "confidential data base." In the case of a notification from a manufacturer or the FDA, the registry responds by notifying patients and their physicians and surgeons. Also provided are updates of their record twice a year (fees: $25 to register; $10 for annual renewals).

Maryland Department of Health and Mental Hygiene

201 West Preston Street

Baltimore, MD 21201

Maryland is the only state to require that surgeons provide women with written information about the advantages, disadvantages, and risks associated with breast implants. This booklet must be given to women at least five days before the operation. Copies are available by writing for *Breast Enlargement: What You Need to Know About Breast Implants.*

National Alliance of Breast Cancer Organizations

1180 Avenue of the Americas
Second Floor
New York, NY 10036
(212) 719-0154

Established in 1986, this nonprofit group of 300 member-organizations describes itself as a central resource for up-to-date information about breast cancer and has also acted as an advocate for breast cancer survivors at all levels of government.

National Cancer Institute

Office of Cancer Communications
Building 31, Room 10a-24
9000 Rockville Pike
Bethesda, MD 20892
(800) 4-CANCER

An institute of the National Institutes of Health, under the U.S. Public Health Service, NCI answers requests for information through its national toll-free telephone number listed above.

National Women's Health Network

1325 G Street, NW
Lower Level
Washington, DC 20005
(202) 347-1140

Established in 1975, this group describes itself as an advocate for improved federal health policies for women. The network makes available educational material on women's health concerns, operates a speaker's bureau and a women's health clearinghouse, and conducts meetings and conferences. It provides information packets on breast implants for a $10 donation to cover postage and photocopying.

National Women's Health Resource Center

2440 M Street, NW, Suite 325
Washington, DC 20037
(202) 293-6045

A national organization devoted to the health of women, its services include a range of clinical, educational, research, and support programs.

Public Citizen Health Research Group
2000 P Street, NW, Suite 700
Washington, DC 20036
(202) 833-3000

This Ralph Nader–founded group was created to perform consumer advocacy work in the areas of health care delivery; occupational safety; and food, drug, and medical device safety. The group conducts research and publishes guides for consumers. It also provides a free information packet on implants for consumers that includes articles and testimony, among other helpful information.

United Scleroderma Foundation
P.O. Box 399
Watsonville, CA 95077
(408) 728-2202
(800) 722-4673

Founded in 1975, this group provides information to people with scleroderma (an autoimmune disorder in which the body's immune system attacks its own tissues) through informational literature, newsletters, physician referrals, and workshops.

**Y-ME National Organization for Breast Cancer
Information and Support**
18220 Harwood Avenue
Homewood, IL 60430
National hotline (outside Chicago): (800) 221-2141
Chicago hotline: (708) 799-8228

A nonprofit organization founded in 1978 by two mastectomy patients, Y-ME provides information and ongoing peer support for patients in all stages of breast disease. The program answers general questions about breast cancer, treatment options, side effects, and general coping mechanisms. Its services include a telephone hotline, one-on-one counseling, educational meetings, referrals, in-service programs for professionals, early detection workshops for the general public, and a wig and prosthesis bank. Pertinent informational brochures are mailed free of charge.

INDEX

Index

About the Authors

Randolph H. Guthrie, M.D., F.A.C.S., after graduating from The Harvard Medical School, completed a full course of training in both general surgery and plastic surgery at Columbia and Cornell Universities and is board certified in the two fields. He has written more than fifty articles in medical journals and books and is the author of one of the leading textbooks on all aspects of breast surgery. While Chief of Plastic Surgery at Memorial Sloan-Kettering Cancer Center, he pioneered the surgery to reconstruct breasts after mastectomies. He is presently a full Professor of Surgery at Cornell University Medical College, an Attending Surgeon at The New York Hospital – Cornell Medical Center, and the Chief of Plastic Surgery at Cornell's New York Downtown Hospital. A long-time crusader against the use of silicone gel-filled implants, as well as some of the more dangerous breast surgical procedures, he has appeared on such shows as "Today," "Nova," and "Nightwatch." He is the President of Save Venice, Inc., the American committee under UNESCO that is charged with restoring the art and architecture of Venice, Italy.

Doug Podolsky is a senior writer at U.S. *News & World Report* where he covers health, medicine, fitness, and nutrition. Prior to that, he was a senior editor at *American Health* magazine. In 1993, he received a Howard W. Blakeslee Award from the American Heart Association for outstanding science journalism.